W0259680

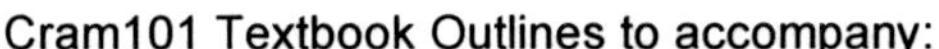

Cram101 Textbook Outlines to accompany:

# Lishmans Organic Psychiatry : A Textbook of Neuropsychiatry

Antony David, 1st Edition

A Content Technologies Inc. publication (c) 2012.

Cram101 Textbook Outlines and Cram101.com are Cram101 Inc. publications and services. All notes, highlights, reviews, and practice tests are written and prepared by Content Technologies and Cram101, all rights reserved.

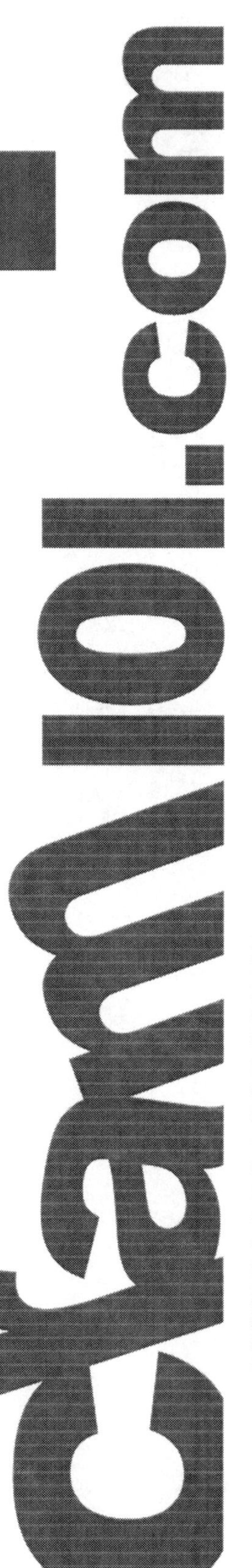

## WHY STOP HERE... THERE'S MORE ONLINE

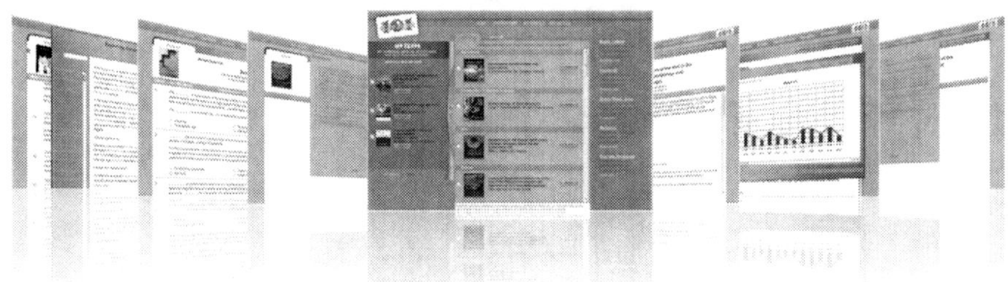

With technology and experience, we've developed tools that make studying easier and efficient. Like this Craml0l textbook notebook, **Craml0l.com** offers you the highlights from every chapter of your actual textbook. However, unlike this notebook, **Craml0l.com** gives you practice tests for each of the chapters. You also get access to in-depth reference material for writing essays and papers.

By purchasing this book, you get 50% off the normal subscription free!. Just enter the promotional code **'DK73DW16488'** on the Cram101.com registration screen.

## CRAMI0I.COM FEATURES:

**Outlines & Highlights**
Just like the ones in this notebook, but with links to additional information.

**Integrated Note Taking**
Add your class notes to the Cram101 notes, print them and maximize your study time.

**Problem Solving**
Step-by-step walk throughs for math, stats and other disciplines.

**Practice Exams**
Five different test taking formats for every chapter.

**Easy Access**
Study any of your books, on any computer, anywhere.

**Unlimited Textbooks**
All the features above for virtually all your textbooks, just add them to your account at no additional cost.

## *TRY THE FIRST CHAPTER FREE!*

Be sure to use the promo code above when registering on Craml0l.com to get 50% off your membership fees.

## STUDYING MADE EASY

This Craml0l notebook is designed to make studying easier and increase your comprehension of the textbook material. Instead of starting with a blank notebook and trying to write down everything discussed in class lectures, you can use this Craml0l textbook notebook and annotate your notes along with the lecture.

***Our goal is to give you the best tools for success.***

For a supreme understanding of the course, pair your notebook with our online tools. Should you decide you prefer Craml0l.com as your study tool,

***we'd like to offer you a trade...***

Our Trade In program is a simple way for us to keep our promise and provide you the best studying tools, regardless of where you purchased your Craml0l textbook notebook. As long as your notebook is in *Like New Condition**, you can send it back to us and we will immediately give you a Craml0l.com account free for 120 days!

## Let The **Trade In** Begin!

### THREE SIMPLE STEPS TO TRADE:

**1.** Go to www.cram101.com/tradein and fill out the packing slip information.

**2.** Submit and print the packing slip and mail it in with your Craml0l textbook notebook.

**3.** Activate your account after you receive your email confirmation.

* Books must be returned in *Like New Condition*, meaning there is no damage to the book including, but not limited to; ripped or torn pages, markings or writing on pages, or folded / creased pages. Upon receiving the book, Craml0l will inspect it and reserves the right to terminate your free Craml0l.com account and return your textbook notebook at the owners expense.

## Learning System

Cram101 Textbook Outlines is a learning system. The notes in this book are the highlights of your textbook, you will never have to highlight a book again.

**How to use this book.** Take this book to class, it is your notebook for the lecture. The notes and highlights on the left hand side of the pages follow the outline and order of the textbook. All you have to do is follow along while your instructor presents the lecture. Circle the items emphasized in class and add other important information on the right side. With Cram101 Textbook Outlines you'll spend less time writing and more time listening. Learning becomes more efficient.

## Cram101.com Online

Increase your studying efficiency by using Cram101.com's practice tests and online reference material. It is the perfect complement to Cram101 Textbook Outlines. Use self-teaching matching tests or simulate in-class testing with comprehensive multiple choice tests, or simply use Cram's true and false tests for quick review. Cram101.com even allows you to enter your in-class notes for an integrated studying format combining the textbook notes with your class notes.

Visit **www.Cram101.com**, click Sign Up at the top of the screen, and enter **DK73DW16488** in the promo code box on the registration screen. Your access to www.Cram101.com is discounted by 50% because you have purchased this book. Sign up and stop highlighting textbooks forever.

Copyright © 2011 by Cram101, Inc. All rights reserved. "Cram101"® and "Never Highlight a Book Again!"® are registered trademarks of Cram101, Inc. ISBN(s): 9781614612605. PUBR-1.201146

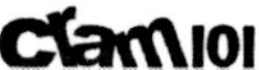

Lishmans Organic Psychiatry : A Textbook of Neuropsychiatry
Antony David, 1st

# CONTENTS

## Chapter 1. Basic Concepts in Neuropsychiatry,

| | |
|---|---|
| Aphasia | Aphasia meaning speechless, is an acquired language disorder in which there is an impairment of any language modality. This may include difficulty in producing or comprehending spoken or written language.<br><br>Traditionally, aphasia suggests the total impairment of language ability, and dysphasia a degree of impairment less than total. |
| Neuropsychiatry | Neuropsychiatry is the branch of medicine dealing with mental disorders attributable to diseases of the nervous system. It preceded the current disciplines of psychiatry and neurology, inasmuch as psychiatrists and neurologists had a common training (Yudofsky and Hales, 2002). However, neurology and psychiatry subsequently split apart and are typically practiced separately. |
| Chronic | In medicine, a chronic disease is a disease that is long-lasting or recurrent. The term chronic describes the course of the disease, or its rate of onset and development. A chronic course is distinguished from a recurrent course; recurrent diseases relapse repeatedly, with periods of remission in between. As an adjective, chronic can refer to a persistent and lasting medical condition. Chronicity is usually applied to a condition that lasts more than three months. The opposite of chronic is acute. |
| Tower of London Test | The Tower of London test is a well-known test used in applied clinical neuropsychology for the assessment of executive functioning specifically to detect deficits in planning, which may occur due to a variety of medical and neuropsychiatric conditions. It is related to the classic problem-solving puzzle known as the Tower of Hanoi.<br><br>The test consists of two boards with pegs and several beads with different colors. |
| Delusion | A delusion is a fixed belief that is either false, fanciful, or derived from deception. In psychiatry, it is defined to be a belief that is pathological (the result of an illness or illness process) and is held despite evidence to the contrary. As a pathology, it is distinct from a belief based on false or incomplete information, dogma, stupidity, apperception, illusion, or other effects of perception. |

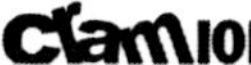





Go to **Cram101.com** for Interactive Practice Exams for this book or virtually any of your books.
And, **NEVER** highlight a book again!

| | |
|---|---|
| Hallucination | A hallucination, in the broadest sense of the word, is a perception in the absence of a stimulus. In a stricter sense, hallucinations are defined as perceptions in a conscious and awake state in the absence of external stimuli which have qualities of real perception, in that they are vivid, substantial, and located in external objective space. The latter definition distinguishes hallucinations from the related phenomena of dreaming, which does not involve wakefulness; illusion, which involves distorted or misinterpreted real perception; imagery, which does not mimic real perception and is under voluntary control; and pseudohallucination, which does not mimic real perception, but is not under voluntary control. |
| Diagnostic and Statistical Manual of Mental Disorders | The Diagnostic and Statistical Manual of Mental Disorders is published by the American Psychiatric Association and provides a common language and standard criteria for the classification of mental disorders. It is used in the United States and in varying degrees around the world, by clinicians, researchers, psychiatric drug regulation agencies, health insurance companies, pharmaceutical companies, and policy makers.<br><br>The DSM has attracted controversy and criticism as well as praise. |
| Mental Disorder | A mental disorder is a psychological or behavioral pattern generally associated with subjective distress or disability that occurs in an individual, and which is not a part of normal development or culture. The recognition and understanding of mental health conditions has changed over time and across cultures, and there are still variations in the definition, assessment, and classification of mental disorders, although standard guideline criteria are widely accepted. A few mental disorders are diagnosed based on the harm to others, regardless of the subject's perception of distress. |
| Delirium | Delirium is a common and severe neuropsychiatric syndrome with core features of acute onset and fluctuating course, attentional deficits and generalized severe disorganization of behavior. It typically involves other cognitive deficits, changes in arousal (hyperactive, hypoactive, or mixed), perceptual deficits, altered sleep-wake cycle, and psychotic features such as hallucinations and delusions. It is often caused by a disease process 'outside' the brain, such as common forms of infection (UTI, pneumonia) or by drug effects, particularly anticholinergic or other CNS depressants (benzodiazepines and opioids). |
| Delirium tremens | Delirium tremens is an acute episode of delirium that is usually caused by withdrawal from alcohol, first described in 1813. Benzodiazepines are the treatment of choice for delirium tremens. |

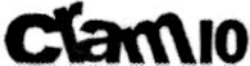





Go to **Cram101.com** for Interactive Practice Exams for this book or virtually any of your books.
And, **NEVER** highlight a book again!

Withdrawal from sedative-hypnotics other than alcohol, such as benzodiazepines or barbiturates can also result in seizures, Delirium tremens and death if not properly managed. Withdrawal from other drugs which are not sedative-hypnotics, such as opioids, marijuana, cocaine etc.

**Differential diagnosis**

A differential diagnosis is a systematic method used to identify unknowns. This method, essentially a process of elimination, is used by taxonomists to identify living organisms, and by physicians, nurse practitioners, physician assistants, and other trained medical professionals to diagnose the specific disease in a patient.

Not all medical diagnoses are differential ones: some diagnoses merely name a set of signs and symptoms that may have more than one possible cause, and some diagnoses are based on intuition or estimations of likelihood. In some cases, there will remain no diagnosis; this suggests the physician has made an error, or that the true diagnosis is unknown to medicine. Removing diagnoses from the list is done by making observations and using tests that should have different results, depending on which diagnosis is correct.

**Synapse**

In the nervous system, a synapse is a junction that permits a neuron to pass an electrical or chemical signal to another cell (neural or otherwise). The word "synapse" comes from "synaptein", which Sir Charles Scott Sherrington and colleagues coined from the Greek "syn-" ("together") and "haptein" ("to clasp").

Synapses are essential to neuronal function: neurons are cells that are specialized to pass signals to individual target cells, and synapses are the means by which they do so.

**Dementia**

Dementia is a serious loss of cognitive ability in a previously unimpaired person, beyond what might be expected from normal aging. It may be static, the result of a unique global brain injury, or progressive, resulting in long-term decline due to damage or disease in the body. Although dementia is far more common in the geriatric population, it may occur in any stage of adulthood.

**Causality**

Causality is the relationship between an event (the cause) and a second event (the effect), where the second event is understood as a consequence of the first.

Go to **Cram101.com** for Interactive Practice Exams for this book or virtually any of your books.
And, **NEVER** highlight a book again!

Though the causes and effects are typically related to changes or events, candidates include objects, processes, properties, variables, facts, and states of affairs; characterizing the causal relationship can be the subject of much debate.

Amnesia

Amnesia is a condition in which memory is disturbed or lost. The causes of amnesia have traditionally been divided into categories. Functional causes are psychological factors, such as mental disorder, post-traumatic stress or, in psychoanalytic terms, defense mechanisms.

Antidepressant

An antidepressant is a psychiatric medication used to alleviate mood disorders, such as major depression and dysthymia and anxiety disorders such as social anxiety disorder. According to Gelder, Mayou '*Geddes (2005) people with a depressive illness will experience a therapeutic effect to their mood, however this will not be experienced in healthy individuals. Drugs including the monoamine oxidase inhibitors (MAOIs), tricyclic antidepressants (TCAs), tetracyclic antidepressants (TeCAs), selective serotonin reuptake inhibitors (SSRIs), and serotonin-norepinephrine reuptake inhibitors (SNRIs) are most commonly associated with the term. These medications are among those most commonly prescribed by psychiatrists and other physicians, and their effectiveness and adverse effects are the subject of many studies and competing claims. Many drugs produce an antidepressant effect, but restrictions on their use have caused controversy and off-label prescription a risk, despite claims of superior efficacy.

Speech disorder

Speech disorders or speech impediments are a type of communication disorders where 'normal' speech is disrupted. This can mean stuttering, lisps, etc. Someone who is unable to speak due to a speech disorder is considered mute.

Brainstem

In vertebrate anatomy the brainstem is the posterior part of the brain, adjoining and structurally continuous with the spinal cord. The brain stem provides the main motor and sensory innervation to the face and neck via the cranial nerves. Though small, this is an extremely important part of the brain as the nerve connections of the motor and sensory systems from the main part of the brain to the rest of the body pass through the brain stem.

Corpus callosum

The corpus callosum is a wide, flat bundle of neural fibers beneath the cortex in the eutherian brain at the longitudinal fissure. It connects the left and right cerebral hemispheres and facilitates interhemispheric communication. It is the largest white matter structure in the brain, consisting of 200-250 million contralateral axonal projections.

Muteness

Muteness is a kind of speech disorder that causes an inability to speak. The term mute originates from the latin word mutus, for silent.

Causes and variations

Go to **Cram101.com** for Interactive Practice Exams for this book or virtually any of your books.
And, **NEVER** highlight a book again!

| | |
|---|---|
| | Selective mutism is a DSM-IV diagnosis that refers to an anxiety disorder in which people are unable to speak in situations causing social anxiety, but are fluent in speech in more comfortable situations. |
| Herpes simplex | Herpes simplex is a viral disease caused by both herpes simplex virus type 1 (HSV-1) and type 2 (HSV-2). Infection with the herpes virus is categorized into one of several distinct disorders based on the site of infection. Oral herpes, the visible symptoms of which are colloquially called cold sores or fever blisters, infects the face and mouth. |
| Conversion disorder | Conversion disorder is a condition in which patients present with neurological symptoms such as numbness, blindness, paralysis, or fits without a physiological cause. It is thought that these problems arise in response to difficulties in the patient's life, and conversion is considered a psychiatric disorder in the International Statistical Classification of Diseases and Related Health Problems (ICD-10) and Diagnostic and Statistical Manual of Mental Disorders 4th edition (DSM-IV). Formerly known as "hysteria", the disorder has arguably been known for millennia, though it came to greatest prominence at the end of the 19th century, when the neurologists Jean-Martin Charcot and Sigmund Freud and psychiatrist Pierre Janet focused their studies on the subject. |

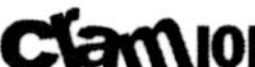





Go to **Cram101.com** for Interactive Practice Exams for this book or virtually any of your books.
And, **NEVER** highlight a book again!

| | |
|---|---|
| Kleine-Levin syndrome | Kleine-Levin Syndrome is a neurological disorder characterized by recurring periods of excessive amounts of sleep and altered behavior. At the onset of an episode the patient becomes drowsy and sleeps for most of the day and night (hypersomnolence), waking only to eat or go to the bathroom. When awake, the patient's whole demeanor is changed, often appearing "spacey" or childlike. |
| Amygdala | The amygdalae are almond-shaped groups of nuclei located deep within the medial temporal lobes of the brain in complex vertebrates, including humans. Shown in research to perform a primary role in the processing and memory of emotional reactions, the amygdalae are considered part of the limbic system. |
| Hypersomnia | Hypersomnia is a disorder characterized by excessive amounts of sleepiness. There are two main categories of hypersomnia: primary hypersomnia and recurrent hypersomnia. Both have the same symptoms but differ in how often they occur. |
| Limbic system | The limbic system is a set of brain structures including the hippocampus, amygdala, anterior thalamic nuclei, septum, limbic cortex and fornix, which seemingly support a variety of functions including emotion, behavior, long term memory, and olfaction. The term "limbic" comes from the Latin limbus, for "border" or "edge". Some scientists have suggested that the concept of the limbic system should be abandoned as obsolete, as it is grounded more in transient tradition than in facts. |
| Amnesia | Amnesia is a condition in which memory is disturbed or lost. The causes of amnesia have traditionally been divided into categories. Functional causes are psychological factors, such as mental disorder, post-traumatic stress or, in psychoanalytic terms, defense mechanisms. |
| Anterograde amnesia | Anterograde amnesia is a loss of the ability to create new memories after the event that caused the amnesia, leading to a partial or complete inability to recall the recent past, while long-term memories from before the event remain intact. Anterograde amnesia and retrograde amnesia, where memories created prior to the event are lost, can occur together in the same patient. To a large degree, anterograde amnesia remains a mysterious ailment because the precise mechanism of storing memories is not yet well understood, although it is known which regions of the brain are involved. |
| Dementia | Dementia is a serious loss of cognitive ability in a previously unimpaired person, beyond what might be expected from normal aging. It may be static, the result of a unique global brain injury, or progressive, resulting in long-term decline due to damage or disease in the body. Although dementia is far more common in the geriatric population, it may occur in any stage of adulthood. |

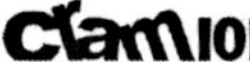





Go to **Cram101.com** for Interactive Practice Exams for this book or virtually any of your books.
And, **NEVER** highlight a book again!

Long-term potentiation

In neuroscience, long-term potentiation is a long-lasting enhancement in signal transmission between two neurons that results from stimulating them synchronously. It is one of several phenomena underlying synaptic plasticity, the ability of chemical synapses to change their strength. As memories are thought to be encoded by modification of synaptic strength, Long term potentiation is widely considered one of the major cellular mechanisms that underlies learning and memory.

Transient epileptic amnesia

Transient epileptic amnesia is a rare but probably underdiagnosed neurological condition which manifests as relatively brief and generally recurring episodes of amnesia caused by underlying temporal lobe epilepsy. Though descriptions of the condition are based on fewer than 100 cases published in the medical literature, and the largest single study to date included 50 people with Transient epileptic amnesia, Transient epileptic amnesia offers considerable theoretical significance as competing theories of human memory attempt to reconcile its implications.

Symptoms

A person experiencing a Transient epileptic amnesia episode has very little short-term memory, so that there is profound difficulty remembering events in the past few minutes (anterograde amnesia), or of events in the hours prior to the onset of the attack, and even memories of important events in recent years may not be accessible during the amnestic event (retrograde amnesia).

Transient global amnesia

Transient global amnesia is "one of the most striking syndromes in clinical neurology" whose key defining characteristic is temporary but almost total disruption of short-term memory with a range of problems accessing older memories. A person in a state of Transient global amnesia exhibits no other signs of impaired cognitive functioning but recalls only the last few moments of consciousness plus deeply-encoded facts of the individual's past, such as his or her own name.

Symptoms

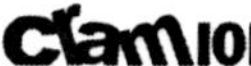





Go to **Cram101.com** for Interactive Practice Exams for this book or virtually any of your books.
And, **NEVER** highlight a book again!

A person having an attack of Transient global amnesia has almost no capacity to establish new memories, but generally appears otherwise mentally alert and lucid, possessing full knowledge of self-identity and identity of close family, and maintaining intact perceptual skills and a wide repertoire of complex learned behavior.

**Alcohol abuse**

Alcohol abuse, as described in the DSM-IV, is a psychiatric diagnosis describing the recurring use of alcoholic beverages despite negative consequences. Alcohol abuse is sometimes referred to by the less specific term alcoholism. However, many definitions of alcoholism exist, and only some are compatible with alcohol abuse.

**Atrophy**

Atrophy is the partial or complete wasting away of a part of the body. Causes of atrophy include mutations (which can destroy the gene to build up the organ), poor nourishment, poor circulation, loss of hormonal support, loss of nerve supply to the target organ, disuse or lack of exercise or disease intrinsic to the tissue itself. Hormonal and nerve inputs that maintain an organ or body part are referred to as trophic [noun] in medical practice. Trophic describes the trophic condition of tissue. A diminished muscular trophic is designated as atrophy.

**Implicit memory**

Implicit memory is a type of memory in which previous experiences aid in the performance of a task without conscious awareness of these previous experiences. Evidence for implicit memory arises in priming, a process whereby subjects show improved performance on tasks for which they have been subconsciously prepared. Implicit memory also leads to the illusion-of-truth effect, which suggests that subjects are more likely to rate as true statements those that they have already heard, regardless of their veracity.

**Priming**

Priming is the implicit memory effect in which exposure to a stimulus influences response to a later stimulus. It can occur following perceptual, semantic, or conceptual stimulus repetition. It happens, for example, that if a person reads a list of words including the word table, and is later asked to complete a word starting with tab, the probability that they will answer table is greater than if not so primed.

**Sense**

Senses are the physiological capacities within organisms that provide inputs for perception. The senses and their operation, classification, and theory are overlapping topics studied by a variety of fields, most notably neuroscience, cognitive psychology (or cognitive science), and philosophy of perception. The nervous system has a specific sensory system or organ, dedicated to each sense.

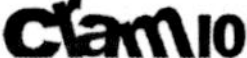





Go to **Cram101.com** for Interactive Practice Exams for this book or virtually any of your books.
And, **NEVER** highlight a book again!

| | |
|---|---|
| Post-concussion syndrome | Post-concussion syndrome, historically called shell shock, is a set of symptoms that a person may experience for weeks, months, or occasionally up to a year or more after a concussion-a mild form of traumatic brain injury . Post concussion syndrome may also occur in moderate and severe cases of traumatic brain injury. Symptoms of Post concussion syndrome, which is the most common entity to be diagnosed in people who have suffered TBI, may occur in 38-80% of mild head injuries. |
| Frontotemporal dementia | Frontotemporal dementia is a clinical syndrome caused by degeneration of the frontal lobe of the brain and may extend back to the temporal lobe. It is one of three syndromes caused by frontotemporal lobar degeneration, and the second most common early-onset dementia after Alzheimer's disease.<br><br>Signs and symptoms<br><br>Symptoms can be classified (roughly) into two groups which underlie the functions of the frontal lobe: behavioural symptoms (and/or personality change) and symptoms related to problems with executive function. |
| Differential diagnosis | A differential diagnosis is a systematic method used to identify unknowns. This method, essentially a process of elimination, is used by taxonomists to identify living organisms, and by physicians, nurse practitioners, physician assistants, and other trained medical professionals to diagnose the specific disease in a patient.<br><br>Not all medical diagnoses are differential ones: some diagnoses merely name a set of signs and symptoms that may have more than one possible cause, and some diagnoses are based on intuition or estimations of likelihood. In some cases, there will remain no diagnosis; this suggests the physician has made an error, or that the true diagnosis is unknown to medicine. Removing diagnoses from the list is done by making observations and using tests that should have different results, depending on which diagnosis is correct. |
| Aphasia | Aphasia meaning speechless, is an acquired language disorder in which there is an impairment of any language modality. This may include difficulty in producing or comprehending spoken or written language. |

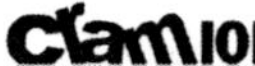





Go to **Cram101.com** for Interactive Practice Exams for this book or virtually any of your books.
And, **NEVER** highlight a book again!

Traditionally, aphasia suggests the total impairment of language ability, and dysphasia a degree of impairment less than total.

Chronic

In medicine, a chronic disease is a disease that is long-lasting or recurrent. The term chronic describes the course of the disease, or its rate of onset and development. A chronic course is distinguished from a recurrent course; recurrent diseases relapse repeatedly, with periods of remission in between. As an adjective, chronic can refer to a persistent and lasting medical condition. Chronicity is usually applied to a condition that lasts more than three months. The opposite of chronic is acute.

Depression

Depression is a state of low mood and aversion to activity that can affect a person's thoughts, behaviour, feelings and physical well-being. It may include feelings of sadness, anxiety, emptiness, hopelessness, worthlessness, guilt, irritability, or restlessness. Depressed people may lose interest in activities that once were pleasurable, experience difficulty concentrating, remembering details, or making decisions, and may contemplate or attempt suicide.

Language disorder

Language disorders or language impairments are disorders that involve the processing of linguistic information. Problems that may be experienced can involve grammar (syntax and/or morphology), semantics (meaning), or other aspects of language. These problems may be receptive (involving impaired language comprehension), expressive (involving language production), or a combination of both.

Schizophrenia

Schizophrenia is a mental disorder characterized by a disintegration of thought processes and of emotional responsiveness. It most commonly manifests as auditory hallucinations, paranoid or bizarre delusions, or disorganized speech and thinking, and it is accompanied by significant social or occupational dysfunction. The onset of symptoms typically occurs in young adulthood, with a global lifetime prevalence of about 0.3-0.7%.

Multi-infarct dementia

Multi-infarct dementia, is one type of vascular dementia. Vascular dementia is the second most common form of dementia after Alzheimer's disease (AD) in older adults. Multi-infarct dementia is thought to be an irreversible form of dementia, and its onset is caused by a number of small strokes or sometimes, one large stroke.

Go to **Cram101.com** for Interactive Practice Exams for this book or virtually any of your books.
And, **NEVER** highlight a book again!

| | |
|---|---|
| Nominal aphasia | Better known around the research community as Anomic aphasia, it is a severe problem with recalling words or names. It is also known as:<br><br>• nominal aphasia<br>• amnesic (or amnestic) aphasia<br><br>Dysnomia refers to a less severe form of this word-recall dysfunction. Learning disabilities caused by name-recall problems are usually diagnosed as dysnomia rather than anomia. |
| Alexia | Alexia is a type of aphasia where damage to the brain causes a patient to lose the ability to read. It is also called word blindness, text blindness or visual aphasia.<br><br>Those who suffer from "alexia" and "dyslexia" can have similar difficulties, however, "alexia" refers to an acquired reading disability, where reading ability had previously been developed, usually occurring in adulthood conditions, while "dyslexia" refers to developmental reading disability. |
| Dyslexia | Dyslexia is a broad term defining a learning disability that impairs a person's fluency or accuracy in being able to read, speak, and spell. and which can manifest itself as a difficulty with phonological awareness, phonological decoding, orthographic coding, auditory short-term memory, and/or rapid naming. Dyslexia is separate and distinct from reading difficulties resulting from other causes, such as a non-neurological deficiency with vision or hearing, or from poor or inadequate reading instruction. |
| Conversion disorder | Conversion disorder is a condition in which patients present with neurological symptoms such as numbness, blindness, paralysis, or fits without a physiological cause. It is thought that these problems arise in response to difficulties in the patient's life, and conversion is considered a psychiatric disorder in the International Statistical Classification of Diseases and Related Health Problems (ICD-10) and Diagnostic and Statistical Manual of Mental Disorders 4th edition (DSM-IV). Formerly known as "hysteria", the disorder has arguably been known for millennia, though it came to greatest prominence at the end of the 19th century, when the neurologists Jean-Martin Charcot and Sigmund Freud and psychiatrist Pierre Janet focused their studies on the subject. |

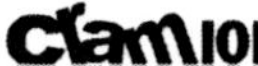





Go to **Cram101.com** for Interactive Practice Exams for this book or virtually any of your books.
And, **NEVER** highlight a book again!

Muteness

Muteness is a kind of speech disorder that causes an inability to speak. The term mute originates from the latin word mutus, for silent.

Causes and variations

Selective mutism is a DSM-IV diagnosis that refers to an anxiety disorder in which people are unable to speak in situations causing social anxiety, but are fluent in speech in more comfortable situations.

Synapse

In the nervous system, a synapse is a junction that permits a neuron to pass an electrical or chemical signal to another cell (neural or otherwise). The word "synapse" comes from "synaptein", which Sir Charles Scott Sherrington and colleagues coined from the Greek "syn-" ("together") and "haptein" ("to clasp").

Synapses are essential to neuronal function: neurons are cells that are specialized to pass signals to individual target cells, and synapses are the means by which they do so.

Apraxia

Apraxia is a disorder caused by damage to specific areas of the cerebrum, characterized by loss of the ability to execute or carry out learned purposeful movements, despite having the desire and the physical ability to perform the movements. It is a disorder of motor planning which may be acquired or developmental, but may not be caused by incoordination, sensory loss, or failure to comprehend simple commands (which can be tested by asking the person to recognize the correct movement from a series). Apraxia should not be confused with ataxia, a lack of coordination of movements, aphasia, an inability to produce and/or comprehend language; abulia, the lack of desire to carry out an action; or allochiria, in which patients perceive stimuli to one side of the body as occurring on the other.

Perception

In philosophy, psychology, and cognitive science, perception is the process of attaining awareness or understanding of sensory information. The word "perception" comes from the Latin words perceptio, percipio, and means "receiving, collecting, action of taking possession, apprehension with the mind or senses."

Go to **Cram101.com** for Interactive Practice Exams for this book or virtually any of your books.
And, **NEVER** highlight a book again!

| | |
|---|---|
| | Perception is one of the oldest fields in psychology. The oldest quantitative law in psychology is the Weber-Fechner law, which quantifies the relationship between the intensity of physical stimuli and their perceptual effects. |
| Gyrus | A gyrus is a ridge on the cerebral cortex. It is generally surrounded by one or more sulci (sl. sulcus). |
| Prosopagnosia | Prosopagnosia is a disorder of face perception where the ability to recognize faces is impaired, while the ability to recognize other objects may be relatively intact. The term originally referred to a condition following acute brain damage, but recently a congenital form of the disorder has been proposed, which may be inherited by about 2.5% of the population. The specific brain area usually associated with prosopagnosia is the fusiform gyrus. |
| Affect | "Affect" is a concept used in philosophy by Spinoza, Deleuze and Guattari. According to Spinoza's Ethics III, 3, Definition 3, an affect is an empowerment, and not a simple change or modification. Affects, according to Deleuze, are not simple affections, as they are independent from their subject. |
| Autism | Autism is a disorder of neural development characterized by impaired social interaction and communication, and by restricted and repetitive behavior. These signs all begin before a child is three years old. Autism affects information processing in the brain by altering how nerve cells and their synapses connect and organize; how this occurs is not well understood. |
| Ganser syndrome | Ganser syndrome is a rare dissociative disorder previously classified as a factitious disorder. It is characterized by nonsensical or wrong answers to questions or doing things incorrectly, other dissociative symptoms such as fugue, amnesia or conversion disorder, often with visual pseudohallucinations and a decreased state of consciousness. It is also sometimes called nonsense syndrome, balderdash syndrome, syndrome of approximate answers, pseudodementia, hysterical pseudodementia or prison psychosis. |
| Tabes dorsalis | Tabes dorsalis is a slow degeneration of the sensory neurons that carry information. The degenerating nerves are in the dorsal columns (posterior columns) of the spinal cord (the portion closest to the back of the body) and carry information that help maintain a person's sense of position (proprioception), vibration, and discriminative touch.<br><br>Cause |

Go to **Cram101.com** for Interactive Practice Exams for this book or virtually any of your books.
And, **NEVER** highlight a book again!

Tabes dorsalis is caused by demyelination secondary to an untreated syphilis infection.

**Dyscalculia**

Dyscalculia is a specific learning disability or difficulty involving innate difficulty in learning or comprehending mathematics. It is akin to dyslexia and can include confusion about math symbols. Dyscalculia can also occur as the result of some types of brain injury.

**Image**

An image is an artifact, for example a two-dimensional picture, that has a similar appearance to some subject--usually a physical object or a person.

Characteristics

Images may be two-dimensional, such as a photograph, screen display, and as well as a three-dimensional, such as a statue or hologram. They may be captured by optical devices--such as cameras, mirrors, lenses, telescopes, microscopes, etc.

**Anosognosia**

Anosognosia is a condition in which a person who suffers disability seems unaware of the existence of his or her disability. Unlike denial, which is a defense mechanism, Anosognosia is rooted in physiology (for example, damage to the frontal or parietal lobe due to illness and disease). This may include unawareness of quite dramatic impairments, such as blindness or paralysis.

**Denial**

Denial is a defense mechanism postulated by Sigmund Freud, in which a person is faced with a fact that is too uncomfortable to accept and rejects it instead, insisting that it is not true despite what may be overwhelming evidence. The subject may use:

- simple denial - deny the reality of the unpleasant fact altogether
- minimisation - admit the fact but deny its seriousness (a combination of denial and rationalisation), or
- projection - admit both the fact and seriousness but deny responsibility.

The concept of denial is particularly important to the study of addiction. The theory of denial was first researched seriously by Anna Freud.

Go to **Cram101.com** for Interactive Practice Exams for this book or virtually any of your books.
And, **NEVER** highlight a book again!

| | |
|---|---|
| Displacement | In Freud's psychology, displacement is an unconscious defense mechanism whereby the mind redirects affects from an object felt to be dangerous or unacceptable to an object felt to be safe or acceptable. For instance, some people punch cushions when they are angry at friends; a college student may snap at his or her roommate when upset about an exam grade.<br><br>Displacement operates in the mind unconsciously and involves emotions, ideas, or wishes being transferred from their original object to a more acceptable substitute. |
| Illusion | An illusion is a distortion of the senses, revealing how the brain normally organizes and interprets sensory stimulation. While illusions distort reality, they are generally shared by most people. Illusions may occur with more of the human senses than vision, but visual illusions, optical illusions, are the most well known and understood. |
| Autoscopy | Autoscopy is the experience in which the individual while believing himself to be awake sees his or her body position outside of his body. Autoscopy comes from the ancient Greek α?τ?ς ("self") and σκοπ?ς ("watcher").<br><br>Autoscopy has intrigued humankind from time immemorial and is abundant in the folklore, mythology, and spiritual narratives of most ancient and modern societies . |
| Experience | Experience as a general concept comprises knowledge of or skill in or observation of some thing or some event gained through involvement in or exposure to that thing or event. The history of the word experience aligns it closely with the concept of experiment.<br><br>The concept of experience generally refers to know-how or procedural knowledge, rather than propositional knowledge: on-the-job training rather than book-learning. |

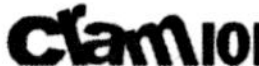





Go to **Cram101.com** for Interactive Practice Exams for this book or virtually any of your books.
And, **NEVER** highlight a book again!

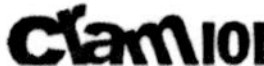



| | |
|---|---|
| Personality disorder | Personality disorders, formerly referred to as character disorders, are a class of personality types and behaviors that the American Psychiatric Association (APA) defines as "an enduring pattern of inner experience and behavior that deviates markedly from the expectations of the culture of the individual who exhibits it". Personality disorders are noted on Axis II of the Diagnostic and Statistical Manual of Mental Disorders or DSM-IV-TR (fourth edition, text revision) of the American Psychiatric Association.<br><br>Personality disorders are also defined by the International Statistical Classification of Diseases and Related Health Problems (ICD-10), which is published by the World Health Organization. |
| Psychosurgery | Psychosurgery is the neurosurgical treatment of mental disorder. It was introduced in 1930s and has a controversial history; Portuguese neurologist Egas Moniz is usually credited with being the originator of psychosurgery, although there had been previous attempts to operate on the brains of mentally ill people. The practice was enthusiastically taken up by American neurologist Walter Freeman who devised his own version of the operation and called it a lobotomy. |

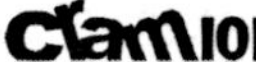





Go to **Cram101.com** for Interactive Practice Exams for this book or virtually any of your books.
And, **NEVER** highlight a book again!

| | |
|---|---|
| Antipsychotic | An antipsychotic is a tranquilizing psychiatric medication primarily used to manage psychosis (including delusions or hallucinations, as well as disordered thought), particularly in schizophrenia and bipolar disorder. A first generation of antipsychotics, known as typical antipsychotics, was discovered in the 1950s. Most of the drugs in the second generation, known as atypical antipsychotics, have been developed more recently, although the first atypical antipsychotic, clozapine, was discovered in the 1950s and introduced clinically in the 1970s. |
| Neuroleptic malignant syndrome | Neuroleptic malignant syndrome is a life- threatening neurological disorder most often caused by an adverse reaction to neuroleptic or antipsychotic drugs. It generally presents with muscle rigidity, fever, autonomic instability and cognitive changes such as delirium, and is associated with elevated creatine phosphokinase (CPK). Incidence of the disease has declined since its discovery (due to changes in prescription habits), but it is still a potential danger to patients being treated with antipsychotics. |
| Neurological examination | A neurological examination is the assessment of sensory neuron and motor responses, especially reflexes, to determine whether the nervous system is impaired. It can be used both as a screening tool and as an investigative tool, the former of which when examining the patient when there is no expected neurological deficit and the latter of which when examining a patient where you do expect to find abnormalities. If a problem is found either in an investigative or screening process then further tests can be carried out to focus on a particular aspect of the nervous system (such as lumbar punctures and blood tests). |
| Dementia | Dementia is a serious loss of cognitive ability in a previously unimpaired person, beyond what might be expected from normal aging. It may be static, the result of a unique global brain injury, or progressive, resulting in long-term decline due to damage or disease in the body. Although dementia is far more common in the geriatric population, it may occur in any stage of adulthood. |
| Dysarthria | Dysarthria is a motor speech disorder resulting from neurological injury, characterized by poor articulation (cf. aphasia: a disorder of the content of speech). Any of the speech subsystems (respiration, phonation, resonance, prosody, and articulation) can be affected. |
| Dysprosody | Dysprosody, which is also known as pseudo-foreign dialect syndrome, refers to a disorder in which one or more of the prosodic functions are either compromised or eliminated completely.<br><br>Prosody refers to the variations in melody, intonation, pauses, stresses, intensity, vocal quality and accents of speech. As a result, prosody has a wide array of functions including expression on linguistic, attitudinal, pragmatic, affective and personal levels of speech. People diagnosed with dysprosody most commonly experience difficulties in pitch or timing control. |

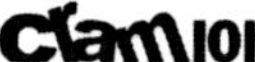





Go to **Cram101.com** for Interactive Practice Exams for this book or virtually any of your books.
And, **NEVER** highlight a book again!

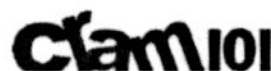



| | |
|---|---|
| Substance abuse | Substance abuse, refers to a maladaptive pattern of use of a substance that is not considered dependent. The term "drug abuse" does not exclude dependency, but is otherwise used in a similar manner in nonmedical contexts. The terms have a huge range of definitions related to taking a psychoactive drug or performance enhancing drug for a non-therapeutic or non-medical effect. |
| Image | An image is an artifact, for example a two-dimensional picture, that has a similar appearance to some subject--usually a physical object or a person.<br><br>Characteristics<br><br>Images may be two-dimensional, such as a photograph, screen display, and as well as a three-dimensional, such as a statue or hologram. They may be captured by optical devices--such as cameras, mirrors, lenses, telescopes, microscopes, etc. |
| Sense | Senses are the physiological capacities within organisms that provide inputs for perception. The senses and their operation, classification, and theory are overlapping topics studied by a variety of fields, most notably neuroscience, cognitive psychology (or cognitive science), and philosophy of perception. The nervous system has a specific sensory system or organ, dedicated to each sense. |
| Anosognosia | Anosognosia is a condition in which a person who suffers disability seems unaware of the existence of his or her disability. Unlike denial, which is a defense mechanism, Anosognosia is rooted in physiology (for example, damage to the frontal or parietal lobe due to illness and disease). This may include unawareness of quite dramatic impairments, such as blindness or paralysis. |
| Euphoria | Euphoria is medically recognized as a mental and emotional state defined as a profound sense of well-being. Technically, euphoria is an affect, but the term is often colloquially used to define emotion as an intense state of transcendent happiness combined with an overwhelming sense of contentment. |

Go to **Cram101.com** for Interactive Practice Exams for this book or virtually any of your books.
And, **NEVER** highlight a book again!

| | |
|---|---|
| | Euphoria is generally considered to be an exaggerated physical and psychological state, sometimes induced by the use of psychoactive drugs and not typically achieved during the normal course of human experience. |
| Hypersomnia | Hypersomnia is a disorder characterized by excessive amounts of sleepiness. There are two main categories of hypersomnia: primary hypersomnia and recurrent hypersomnia. Both have the same symptoms but differ in how often they occur. |
| Wechsler Adult Intelligence Scale | The Wechsler Adult Intelligence Scale intelligence quotient (IQ) tests are the primary clinical instruments used to measure adult and adolescent intelligence. The original Wechsler Adult Intelligence Scale (Form I) was published in February 1955 by David Wechsler, as a revision of the Wechsler-Bellevue Intelligence Scale. The fourth edition of the test (Wechsler Adult Intelligence Scale-IV) was released in 2008 by Pearson. |
| Hallucination | A hallucination, in the broadest sense of the word, is a perception in the absence of a stimulus. In a stricter sense, hallucinations are defined as perceptions in a conscious and awake state in the absence of external stimuli which have qualities of real perception, in that they are vivid, substantial, and located in external objective space. The latter definition distinguishes hallucinations from the related phenomena of dreaming, which does not involve wakefulness; illusion, which involves distorted or misinterpreted real perception; imagery, which does not mimic real perception and is under voluntary control; and pseudohallucination, which does not mimic real perception, but is not under voluntary control. |
| Illusion | An illusion is a distortion of the senses, revealing how the brain normally organizes and interprets sensory stimulation. While illusions distort reality, they are generally shared by most people. Illusions may occur with more of the human senses than vision, but visual illusions, optical illusions, are the most well known and understood. |
| Electroencephalography | Electroencephalography is the recording of electrical activity along the scalp produced by the firing of neurons within the brain. In clinical contexts, EEG refers to the recording of the brain's spontaneous electrical activity over a short period of time, usually 20-40 minutes, as recorded from multiple electrodes placed on the scalp. In neurology, the main diagnostic application of EE is in the case of epilepsy, as epileptic activity can create clear abnormalities on a standard EEG study. |

Go to **Cram101.com** for Interactive Practice Exams for this book or virtually any of your books.
And, **NEVER** highlight a book again!

| | |
|---|---|
| Chlorpromazine | Chlorpromazine is a typical antipsychotic. First synthesized on December 11, 1950, chlorpromazine was the first drug developed with specific antipsychotic action, and would serve as the prototype for the phenothiazine class of drugs, which later grew to comprise several other agents. The introduction of chlorpromazine into clinical use has been described as the single greatest advance in psychiatric care, dramatically improving the prognosis of patients in psychiatric hospitals worldwide; the availability of antipsychotic drugs curtailed indiscriminate use of electroconvulsive therapy and psychosurgery, and was one of the driving forces behind the deinstitutionalization movement. |
| Electroconvulsive therapy | Electroconvulsive therapy also known as electroshock (although the use of this term has generally decreased in use by many professionals due to its negative association with earlier treatment practices), is psychiatric treatment in which seizures are electrically induced in anesthetized patients for therapeutic effect. Today, ECT is most often used as a treatment for severe depression which has not responded to other treatment, and is also used in the treatment of mania (often in bipolar disorder), and catatonia. It was first introduced in the 1930s and gained widespread use as a form of treatment in the 1940s and 1950s; today, an estimated 1 million people worldwide receive ECT every year, usually in a course of 6-12 treatments administered two or three times a week. |
| Event-related potential | An event-related potential is any measured brain response that is directly the result of a thought or perception. More formally, it is any stereotyped electrophysiological response to an internal or external stimulus.<br><br>Event related potentials are measured with electroencephalography (EEG). |
| Aphasia | Aphasia meaning speechless, is an acquired language disorder in which there is an impairment of any language modality. This may include difficulty in producing or comprehending spoken or written language.<br><br>Traditionally, aphasia suggests the total impairment of language ability, and dysphasia a degree of impairment less than total. |

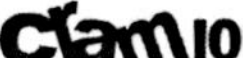





Go to **Cram101.com** for Interactive Practice Exams for this book or virtually any of your books.
And, **NEVER** highlight a book again!

| | |
|---|---|
| Atrophy | Atrophy is the partial or complete wasting away of a part of the body. Causes of atrophy include mutations (which can destroy the gene to build up the organ), poor nourishment, poor circulation, loss of hormonal support, loss of nerve supply to the target organ, disuse or lack of exercise or disease intrinsic to the tissue itself. Hormonal and nerve inputs that maintain an organ or body part are referred to as trophic [noun] in medical practice. Trophic describes the trophic condition of tissue. A diminished muscular trophic is designated as atrophy. |
| Cognitive dysfunction | Cognitive dysfunction is defined as unusually poor mental function, associated with confusion, forgetfulness and difficulty concentrating. A number of medical or psychiatric conditions and treatments can cause such symptoms, including heavy metal poisoning (in particular mercury poisoning), menopause, fibromyalgia, ADHD and sleep disorders (including disrupted sleep). The term brain fog is not commonly used to describe people with dementia or other conditions that are known to cause confusion and memory problems, but it can be used as a synonym for sleep inertia or grogginess upon being awakened from deep sleep. |
| Schizophrenia | Schizophrenia is a mental disorder characterized by a disintegration of thought processes and of emotional responsiveness. It most commonly manifests as auditory hallucinations, paranoid or bizarre delusions, or disorganized speech and thinking, and it is accompanied by significant social or occupational dysfunction. The onset of symptoms typically occurs in young adulthood, with a global lifetime prevalence of about 0.3-0.7%. |
| Kleine-Levin syndrome | Kleine-Levin Syndrome is a neurological disorder characterized by recurring periods of excessive amounts of sleep and altered behavior. At the onset of an episode the patient becomes drowsy and sleeps for most of the day and night (hypersomnolence), waking only to eat or go to the bathroom. When awake, the patient's whole demeanor is changed, often appearing "spacey" or childlike. |
| Attention deficit hyperactivity disorder | Attention deficit hyperactivity disorder is a neurobehavioral developmental disorder. It is primarily characterized by "the co-existence of attentional problems and hyperactivity, with each behavior occurring infrequently alone" and symptoms starting before seven years of age.<br><br>Attention deficit hyperactivity disorder is the most commonly studied and diagnosed psychiatric disorder in children, affecting about 3 to 5 percent of children globally and diagnosed in about 2 to 16 percent of school aged children. |

Go to **Cram101.com** for Interactive Practice Exams for this book or virtually any of your books.
And, **NEVER** highlight a book again!

**Contrast**

Contrast is the difference in visual properties that makes an object (or its representation in an image) distinguishable from other objects and the background. In visual perception of the real world, contrast is determined by the difference in the color and brightness of the object and other objects within the same field of view. Because the human visual system is more sensitive to contrast than absolute luminance, we can perceive the world similarly regardless of the huge changes in illumination over the day or from place to place.

**Hyperactivity**

Hyperactivity can be described as a physical state in which a person is abnormally and easily excitable or exuberant. Strong emotional reactions, impulsive behavior, and sometimes a short span of attention are also typical for a hyperactive person. Some individuals may show these characteristics naturally, as personality differs from person to person. Nonetheless, when hyperactivity starts to become a problem for the person or others, it may be classified as a medical disorder. The slang term "hyper" is used to describe someone who is in a hyperactive state.

**Metabolism**

Metabolism is the set of chemical reactions that happen in living organisms to maintain life. These processes allow organisms to grow and reproduce, maintain their structures, and respond to their environments. Metabolism is usually divided into two categories. Catabolism breaks down organic matter, for example to harvest energy in cellular respiration. Anabolism uses energy to construct components of cells such as proteins and nucleic acids.

**Dopamine**

Dopamine is a catecholamine neurotransmitter present in a wide variety of animals, including both vertebrates and invertebrates. In the brain, this substituted phenethylamine functions as a neurotransmitter, activating the five known types of dopamine receptors--$D_1$, $D_2$, $D_3$, $D_4$, and $D_5$--and their variants. Dopamine is produced in several areas of the brain, including the substantia nigra and the ventral tegmental area.

**Dopamine transporter**

The dopamine transporter is a membrane-spanning protein that pumps the neurotransmitter dopamine out of the synapse back into cytosol, from which other transporters sequester DA and NE into vesicles for later storage and release. Dopamine reuptake via DAT provides the primary mechanism through which dopamine is cleared from synapses except in the prefrontal cortex, where dopamine uptake via the norepinephrine transporter plays that role.

DAT is thought to be implicated in a number of dopamine-related disorders, including attention deficit hyperactivity disorder, bipolar disorder, clinical depression, and alcoholism.

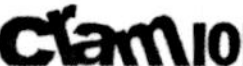





Go to **Cram101.com** for Interactive Practice Exams for this book or virtually any of your books.
And, **NEVER** highlight a book again!

|  |  |
| --- | --- |
| Psychopharmacology | Psychopharmacology is the study of drug-induced changes in mood, sensation, thinking, and behavior.<br><br>The field of psychopharmacology studies a wide range of substances with various types of psychoactive properties. The professional and commercial fields of pharmacology and psychopharmacology do not mainly focus on psychedelic or recreational drugs, as the majority of studies are conducted for the development, study, and use of drugs for the modification of behavior and the alleviation of symptoms, particularly in the treatment of mental disorders (psychiatric medication). |
| Electromyography | Electromyography is a technique for evaluating and recording the electrical activity produced by skeletal muscles. EMG is performed using an instrument called an electromyograph, to produce a record called an electromyogram. An electromyograph detects the electrical potential generated by muscle cells when these cells are electrically or neurologically activated. |
| Scan | SCAN is a set of tools created by WHO aimed at diagnosing and measuring mental illness that may occur in adult life. It is not constructed explicitly for use with either ICD-10 or DSM-IV but can be used for both systems. The SCAN system was originally called PSE, or Present State Examination, but since version 10 (PSE-10), the commonly accepted name has been SCAN. The current version of SCAN is 2.1. |
| Bender-Gestalt Test | The Bender Visual Motor Gestalt Test, or simply the Bender-Gestalt test, is a psychological test first developed by child neuropsychiatrist Lauretta Bender. The test is used to evaluate "visual-motor maturity", to screen for developmental disorders, or to assess neurological function or brain damage.<br><br>The original test consists of nine figures, each on its own 3 × 5 card. |
| Perception | In philosophy, psychology, and cognitive science, perception is the process of attaining awareness or understanding of sensory information. The word "perception" comes from the Latin words perceptio, percipio, and means "receiving, collecting, action of taking possession, apprehension with the mind or senses." |

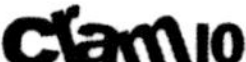





Go to **Cram101.com** for Interactive Practice Exams for this book or virtually any of your books.
And, **NEVER** highlight a book again!

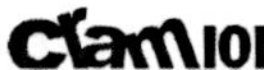



Perception is one of the oldest fields in psychology. The oldest quantitative law in psychology is the Weber-Fechner law, which quantifies the relationship between the intensity of physical stimuli and their perceptual effects.

Pain

Pain is "an unpleasant sensory and emotional experience associated with actual or potential tissue damage, or described in terms of such damage." It is the feeling common to such experiences as stubbing a toe, burning a finger, putting iodine on a cut, and bumping the "funny bone".

Pain motivates us to withdraw from potentially damaging situations, protect a damaged body part while it heals, and avoid those situations in the future. Most pain resolves promptly once the painful stimulus is removed and the body has healed, but sometimes pain persists despite removal of the stimulus and apparent healing of the body; and sometimes pain arises in the absence of any detectable stimulus, damage or disease.

Benton Visual Retention Test

The Benton Visual Retention Test is an individually administered test for ages 8-adult that measures visual perception and visual memory . It can also be used to help identify possible learning disabilities. The child is shown 10 designs, one at a time, and asked to reproduce each one as exactly as possible on plain paper from memory.

Tower of London Test

The Tower of London test is a well-known test used in applied clinical neuropsychology for the assessment of executive functioning specifically to detect deficits in planning, which may occur due to a variety of medical and neuropsychiatric conditions. It is related to the classic problem-solving puzzle known as the Tower of Hanoi.

The test consists of two boards with pegs and several beads with different colors.

Neuropsychological Test

Neuropsychological tests are specifically designed tasks used to measure a psychological function known to be linked to a particular brain structure or pathway. They usually involve the systematic administration of clearly defined procedures in a formal environment. Neuropsychological tests are typically administered to a single person working with an examiner in a quiet office environment, free from distractions.

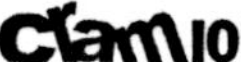





Go to **Cram101.com** for Interactive Practice Exams for this book or virtually any of your books.
And, **NEVER** highlight a book again!

| | |
|---|---|
| Stress | Stress is a term in psychology and biology, first coined in the biological context in the 1930s, which has in more recent decades become commonly used in popular parlance. It refers to the consequence of the failure of an organism - human or animal - to respond appropriately to emotional or physical threats, whether actual or imagined.<br><br>Signs of stress may be cognitive, emotional, physical or behavioral. |
| Visual memory | Visual memory is a part of memory preserving some characteristics of our senses pertaining to visual experience. We are able to place in memory information that resembles objects, places, animals or people in sort of a mental image. Some authors refer to this experience as an "our mind's eye" through which we can retrieve from our memory a mental image of the original object, place, animal or person. |
| Mental Disorder | A mental disorder is a psychological or behavioral pattern generally associated with subjective distress or disability that occurs in an individual, and which is not a part of normal development or culture. The recognition and understanding of mental health conditions has changed over time and across cultures, and there are still variations in the definition, assessment, and classification of mental disorders, although standard guideline criteria are widely accepted. A few mental disorders are diagnosed based on the harm to others, regardless of the subject's perception of distress. |

Go to **Cram101.com** for Interactive Practice Exams for this book or virtually any of your books.
And, **NEVER** highlight a book again!

| | |
|---|---|
| Dementia | Dementia is a serious loss of cognitive ability in a previously unimpaired person, beyond what might be expected from normal aging. It may be static, the result of a unique global brain injury, or progressive, resulting in long-term decline due to damage or disease in the body. Although dementia is far more common in the geriatric population, it may occur in any stage of adulthood. |
| Brain damage | Brain damage is the destruction or degeneration of brain cells. Brain injuries occur due to a wide range of internal and external factors. A common category with the greatest number of injuries is traumatic brain injury (TBI) following physical trauma or head injury from an outside source, and the term acquired brain injury (ABI) is used in appropriate circles, to differentiate brain injuries occurring after birth from injury due to a disorder or congenital malady. |
| Pathophysiology | Pathophysiology is the study of the changes of normal mechanical, physical, and biochemical functions, either caused by a disease, or resulting from an abnormal syndrome. More formally, it is the branch of medicine which deals with any disturbances of body functions, caused by disease or prodromal symptoms.<br><br>An alternative definition is "the study of the biological and physical manifestations of disease as they correlate with the underlying abnormalities and physiological disturbances."<br><br>The study of pathology and the study of pathophysiology often involves substantial overlap in diseases and processes, but pathology emphasizes direct observations, while pathophysiology emphasizes quantifiable measurements. |
| Neuroleptic malignant syndrome | Neuroleptic malignant syndrome is a life- threatening neurological disorder most often caused by an adverse reaction to neuroleptic or antipsychotic drugs. It generally presents with muscle rigidity, fever, autonomic instability and cognitive changes such as delirium, and is associated with elevated creatine phosphokinase (CPK). Incidence of the disease has declined since its discovery (due to changes in prescription habits), but it is still a potential danger to patients being treated with antipsychotics. |
| Torticollis | Torticollis is a stiff neck associated with muscle spasm, classically causing lateral flexion contracture of the cervical spine musculature (a condition in which the head is tilted to one side). The muscles affected are principally those supplied by the spinal accessory nerve. |

Go to **Cram101.com** for Interactive Practice Exams for this book or virtually any of your books.
And, **NEVER** highlight a book again!

| | |
|---|---|
| Kleine-Levin syndrome | Kleine-Levin Syndrome is a neurological disorder characterized by recurring periods of excessive amounts of sleep and altered behavior. At the onset of an episode the patient becomes drowsy and sleeps for most of the day and night (hypersomnolence), waking only to eat or go to the bathroom. When awake, the patient's whole demeanor is changed, often appearing "spacey" or childlike. |
| Hypersomnia | Hypersomnia is a disorder characterized by excessive amounts of sleepiness. There are two main categories of hypersomnia: primary hypersomnia and recurrent hypersomnia. Both have the same symptoms but differ in how often they occur. |
| Substance abuse | Substance abuse, refers to a maladaptive pattern of use of a substance that is not considered dependent. The term "drug abuse" does not exclude dependency, but is otherwise used in a similar manner in nonmedical contexts. The terms have a huge range of definitions related to taking a psychoactive drug or performance enhancing drug for a non-therapeutic or non-medical effect. |
| Aphasia | Aphasia meaning speechless, is an acquired language disorder in which there is an impairment of any language modality. This may include difficulty in producing or comprehending spoken or written language.<br><br>Traditionally, aphasia suggests the total impairment of language ability, and dysphasia a degree of impairment less than total. |
| Reduplicative paramnesia | Reduplicative paramnesia is the delusional belief that a place or location has been duplicated, existing in two or more places simultaneously, or that it has been 'relocated' to another site. It is one of the delusional misidentification syndromes and, although rare, is most commonly associated with acquired brain injury, particularly simultaneous damage to the right cerebral hemisphere and to both frontal lobes.<br><br>History |

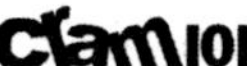





Go to **Cram101.com** for Interactive Practice Exams for this book or virtually any of your books.
And, **NEVER** highlight a book again!

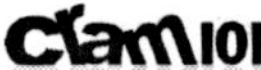



The term reduplicative paramnesia was first used in 1903 by neurologist Arnold Pick to describe a condition in a patient with suspected Alzheimer's disease who insisted that she had been moved from Pick's city clinic, to one she claimed looked identical but was in a familiar suburb.

Chronic

In medicine, a chronic disease is a disease that is long-lasting or recurrent. The term chronic describes the course of the disease, or its rate of onset and development. A chronic course is distinguished from a recurrent course; recurrent diseases relapse repeatedly, with periods of remission in between. As an adjective, chronic can refer to a persistent and lasting medical condition. Chronicity is usually applied to a condition that lasts more than three months. The opposite of chronic is acute.

Post-concussion syndrome

Post-concussion syndrome, historically called shell shock, is a set of symptoms that a person may experience for weeks, months, or occasionally up to a year or more after a concussion-a mild form of traumatic brain injury . Post concussion syndrome may also occur in moderate and severe cases of traumatic brain injury. Symptoms of Post concussion syndrome, which is the most common entity to be diagnosed in people who have suffered TBI, may occur in 38-80% of mild head injuries.

Delirium

Delirium is a common and severe neuropsychiatric syndrome with core features of acute onset and fluctuating course, attentional deficits and generalized severe disorganization of behavior. It typically involves other cognitive deficits, changes in arousal (hyperactive, hypoactive, or mixed), perceptual deficits, altered sleep-wake cycle, and psychotic features such as hallucinations and delusions. It is often caused by a disease process 'outside' the brain, such as common forms of infection (UTI, pneumonia) or by drug effects, particularly anticholinergic or other CNS depressants (benzodiazepines and opioids).

Disability

A disability may be physical, cognitive, mental, sensory, emotional, developmental or some combination of these.
Disabilities is an umbrella term, covering impairments, activity limitations, and participation restrictions. An impairment is a problem in body function or structure; an activity limitation is a difficulty encountered by an individual in executing a task or action; while a participation restriction is a problem experienced by an individual in involvement in life situations.

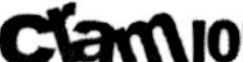





Go to **Cram101.com** for Interactive Practice Exams for this book or virtually any of your books.
And, **NEVER** highlight a book again!

Bromocriptine

Bromocriptine an ergoline derivative, is a dopamine agonist that is used in the treatment of pituitary tumors, Parkinson's disease (PD), hyperprolactinaemia, neuroleptic malignant syndrome, and type 2 diabetes.

Indications

Amenorrhea, female infertility, galactorrhea, hypogonadism, and acromegaly may all be caused by pituitary problems, such as hyperprolactinaemia, and therefore, these problems may be treated by this drug. In 2009, bromocriptine mesylate was approved by the FDA for treatment of type 2 diabetes under the trade name Cycloset (VeroScience).

Dopamine

Dopamine is a catecholamine neurotransmitter present in a wide variety of animals, including both vertebrates and invertebrates. In the brain, this substituted phenethylamine functions as a neurotransmitter, activating the five known types of dopamine receptors--$D_1$, $D_2$, $D_3$, $D_4$, and $D_5$--and their variants. Dopamine is produced in several areas of the brain, including the substantia nigra and the ventral tegmental area.

Dopamine agonist

A dopamine agonist is a compound that activates dopamine receptors in the absence of dopamine. Dopamine agonists activate signaling pathways through the dopamine receptor and trimeric G-proteins, ultimately leading to changes in gene transcription.

Uses

Some medical drugs act as dopamine agonists and can treat hypodopaminergic (low dopamine) conditions; they are typically used for treating Parkinson's disease and certain pituitary tumors (prolactinoma), and may be useful for restless legs syndrome (RLS).

Mood disorder

Mood disorder is the term designating a group of diagnoses in the Diagnostic and Statistical Manual of Mental Disorders (DSM IV TR) classification system where a disturbance in the person's mood is hypothesized to be the main underlying feature. The classification is known as mood (affective) disorders in ICD 10.

Go to **Cram101.com** for Interactive Practice Exams for this book or virtually any of your books.
And, **NEVER** highlight a book again!

English psychiatrist Henry Maudsley proposed an overarching category of affective disorder.

Anxiety

Anxiety is a psychological and physiological state characterized by somatic, emotional, cognitive, and behavioral components. The root meaning of the word anxiety is 'to vex or trouble'; in either the absence or presence of psychological stress, anxiety can create feelings of fear, worry, uneasiness and dread. Anxiety is considered to be a normal reaction to stress.

Anxiety disorder

Anxiety disorders are blanket terms covering several different forms of abnormal and pathological fear and anxiety which only came under the aegis of psychiatry at the very end of the 19th century. Gelder, Mayou ' Geddes (2005) explains that anxiety disorders are classified in two groups: continuous symptoms and episodic symptoms. Current psychiatric diagnostic criteria recognize a wide variety of anxiety disorders.

Depression

Depression is a state of low mood and aversion to activity that can affect a person's thoughts, behaviour, feelings and physical well-being. It may include feelings of sadness, anxiety, emptiness, hopelessness, worthlessness, guilt, irritability, or restlessness. Depressed people may lose interest in activities that once were pleasurable, experience difficulty concentrating, remembering details, or making decisions, and may contemplate or attempt suicide.

Phobia

A phobia is an irrational, intense and persistent fear of certain situations, activities, things, animals, or people. The main symptom of this disorder is the excessive and unreasonable desire to avoid the feared stimulus. When the fear is beyond one's control, and if the fear is interfering with daily life, then a diagnosis under one of the anxiety disorders can be made.

Agoraphobia

Agoraphobia is an anxiety disorder. Agoraphobia may arise by the fear of having a panic attack in a setting from which there is no perceived easy means of escape. Alternatively, social anxiety problems may also be an underlying cause.

Stress

Stress is a term in psychology and biology, first coined in the biological context in the 1930s, which has in more recent decades become commonly used in popular parlance. It refers to the consequence of the failure of an organism - human or animal - to respond appropriately to emotional or physical threats, whether actual or imagined.

Signs of stress may be cognitive, emotional, physical or behavioral.

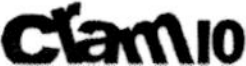





Go to **Cram101.com** for Interactive Practice Exams for this book or virtually any of your books.
And, **NEVER** highlight a book again!

| | |
|---|---|
| Ganser syndrome | Ganser syndrome is a rare dissociative disorder previously classified as a factitious disorder. It is characterized by nonsensical or wrong answers to questions or doing things incorrectly, other dissociative symptoms such as fugue, amnesia or conversion disorder, often with visual pseudohallucinations and a decreased state of consciousness. It is also sometimes called nonsense syndrome, balderdash syndrome, syndrome of approximate answers, pseudodementia, hysterical pseudodementia or prison psychosis. |
| Traumatic brain injury | Traumatic brain injury occurs when an external force traumatically injures the brain. Traumatic brain injury can be classified based on severity, mechanism (closed or penetrating head injury), or other features (e.g. occurring in a specific location or over a widespread area). Head injury usually refers to Traumatic brain injury, but is a broader category because it can involve damage to structures other than the brain, such as the scalp and skull. |
| Differential diagnosis | A differential diagnosis is a systematic method used to identify unknowns. This method, essentially a process of elimination, is used by taxonomists to identify living organisms, and by physicians, nurse practitioners, physician assistants, and other trained medical professionals to diagnose the specific disease in a patient.<br><br>Not all medical diagnoses are differential ones: some diagnoses merely name a set of signs and symptoms that may have more than one possible cause, and some diagnoses are based on intuition or estimations of likelihood. In some cases, there will remain no diagnosis; this suggests the physician has made an error, or that the true diagnosis is unknown to medicine. Removing diagnoses from the list is done by making observations and using tests that should have different results, depending on which diagnosis is correct. |
| Diogenes syndrome | Diogenes syndrome, is a disorder characterized by extreme self-neglect, domestic squalor, social withdrawal, apathy, compulsive hoarding of rubbish, and lack of shame.<br><br>The condition was first recognized in 1966 and designated Diogenes syndrome by Clark et al. Not only did he not hoard, but he actually sought human company by venturing daily to the Agora. Therefore, this eponym is considered to be a misnomer. |
| Community | In biological terms, a community is a group of interacting organisms sharing a populated environment. In human communities, intent, belief, resources, preferences, needs, risks, and a number of other conditions may be present and common, affecting the identity of the participants and their degree of cohesiveness. |

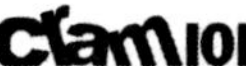





Go to **Cram101.com** for Interactive Practice Exams for this book or virtually any of your books.
And, **NEVER** highlight a book again!

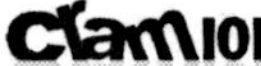



| | |
|---|---|
| Catecholamine | Catecholamines are "fight-or-flight" hormones released by the adrenal glands in response to stress. They are part of the sympathetic nervous system.<br><br>They are called catecholamines because they contain a catechol or 3,4-dihydroxylphenyl group. |
| Pharmacotherapy | Pharmacotherapy is the treatment of disease through the administration of drugs. As such, it is considered part of the larger category of therapy.<br><br>Pharmacists are experts in pharmacotherapy and are responsible for ensuring the safe, appropriate, and economical use of medicines. As pharmacotherapy specialists, pharmacists have responsibility for direct patient care, often functioning as a member of a multidisciplinary team, and acting as the primary source of drug-related information for other healthcare professionals. |
| Citalopram | Citalopram is an antidepressant drug of the selective serotonin reuptake inhibitor (SSRI) class. It has U.S. Food and Drug Administration (FDA) approval to treat major depression, and is prescribed off-label for a number of anxiety conditions.<br><br>History<br><br>Citalopram was originally created in 1989 by the pharmaceutical company Lundbeck. |
| Selective serotonin reuptake inhibitor | Selective serotonin reuptake inhibitors or serotonin-specific reuptake inhibitor are a class of compounds typically used as antidepressants in the treatment of depression, anxiety disorders, and some personality disorders. They are also typically effective and used in treating some cases of insomnia. |

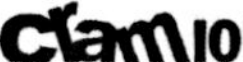





Go to **Cram101.com** for Interactive Practice Exams for this book or virtually any of your books.
And, **NEVER** highlight a book again!

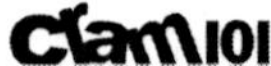



Selective serotonin reuptake inhibitors are believed to increase the extracellular level of the neurotransmitter serotonin by inhibiting its reuptake into the presynaptic cell, increasing the level of serotonin in the synaptic cleft available to bind to the postsynaptic receptor.

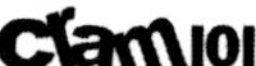





Go to **Cram101.com** for Interactive Practice Exams for this book or virtually any of your books.
And, **NEVER** highlight a book again!

| | |
|---|---|
| Amnesia | Amnesia is a condition in which memory is disturbed or lost. The causes of amnesia have traditionally been divided into categories. Functional causes are psychological factors, such as mental disorder, post-traumatic stress or, in psychoanalytic terms, defense mechanisms. |
| Dementia | Dementia is a serious loss of cognitive ability in a previously unimpaired person, beyond what might be expected from normal aging. It may be static, the result of a unique global brain injury, or progressive, resulting in long-term decline due to damage or disease in the body. Although dementia is far more common in the geriatric population, it may occur in any stage of adulthood. |
| Corpus callosum | The corpus callosum is a wide, flat bundle of neural fibers beneath the cortex in the eutherian brain at the longitudinal fissure. It connects the left and right cerebral hemispheres and facilitates interhemispheric communication. It is the largest white matter structure in the brain, consisting of 200-250 million contralateral axonal projections. |
| Prolactin | Prolactin is a protein that in humans is encoded by the PRL gene. Prolactin is a peptide hormone discovered by Dr. Henry Friesen, primarily associated with lactation. In breastfeeding, the act of an infant suckling the nipple stimulates the production of oxytocin, which stimulates the "milk let-down" reflex, which fills the breast with milk via a process called lactogenesis, in preparation for the next feed. |
| Medical error | Medical error is may be defined as a preventable adverse effect of care, whether or not it is evident or harmful to the patient. This might include an inaccurate or incomplete diagnosis or treatment of a disease, injury, syndromem behavior, infection, or other ailment. As a general acceptance, a medical error occurs when a health-care provider chose an inappropriate method of care or the health provider chose the right solution of care but executed it incorrectly. Medical errors are often described as human errors in healthcare. |
| Cognitive dysfunction | Cognitive dysfunction is defined as unusually poor mental function, associated with confusion, forgetfulness and difficulty concentrating. A number of medical or psychiatric conditions and treatments can cause such symptoms, including heavy metal poisoning (in particular mercury poisoning), menopause, fibromyalgia, ADHD and sleep disorders (including disrupted sleep). The term brain fog is not commonly used to describe people with dementia or other conditions that are known to cause confusion and memory problems, but it can be used as a synonym for sleep inertia or grogginess upon being awakened from deep sleep. |

Go to **Cram101.com** for Interactive Practice Exams for this book or virtually any of your books.
And, **NEVER** highlight a book again!

| | |
|---|---|
| Dissociative disorder | Dissociative disorders are defined as conditions that involve disruptions or breakdowns of memory, awareness, identity and/or perception. The hypothesis is that symptoms can result, to the extent of interfering with a person's general functioning, when one or more of these functions is disrupted.<br><br>The five dissociative disorders listed in the DSM IV are as follows:<br><br>• Depersonalization disorder (DSM-IV Codes 300.6) - periods of detachment from self or surrounding which may be experienced as "unreal" (lacking in control of or "outside of" self) while retaining awareness that this is only a feeling and not a reality.<br>• Dissociative amnesia (DSM-IV Codes 300.12) (formerly Psychogenic Amnesia) - noticeable impairment of recall resulting from emotional trauma<br>• Dissociative fugue (DSM-IV Codes 300.13) (formerly Psychogenic Fugue) - physical desertion of familiar surroundings and experience of impaired recall of the past. |
| Palliative care | Palliative care is any form of medical care or treatment that concentrates on reducing the severity of disease symptoms, rather than striving to halt, delay, or reverse progression of the disease itself or provide a cure. The goal is to prevent and relieve suffering and to improve quality of life for people facing serious, complex illness. Unlike hospice, palliative care is not dependent on prognosis and is offered in conjunction with curative and all other appropriate forms of medical treatment. |
| Ganser syndrome | Ganser syndrome is a rare dissociative disorder previously classified as a factitious disorder. It is characterized by nonsensical or wrong answers to questions or doing things incorrectly, other dissociative symptoms such as fugue, amnesia or conversion disorder, often with visual pseudohallucinations and a decreased state of consciousness. It is also sometimes called nonsense syndrome, balderdash syndrome, syndrome of approximate answers, pseudodementia, hysterical pseudodementia or prison psychosis. |
| Progressive supranuclear palsy | Progressive supranuclear palsy (or the Steele-Richardson-Olszewski syndrome, after the Canadian physicians who described it in 1963) is a rare degenerative disease involving the gradual deterioration and death of selected areas of the brain. |

Go to **Cram101.com** for Interactive Practice Exams for this book or virtually any of your books.
And, **NEVER** highlight a book again!

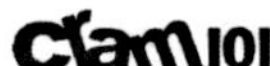



Males and females are affected approximately equally and there is no racial, geographical or occupational predilection. Approximately 6 people per 100,000 population have Progressive supranuclear palsy.

It has been described as a tauopathy.

Tamoxifen

Tamoxifen is an antagonist of the estrogen receptor in breast tissue via its active metabolite, hydroxytamoxifen. In other tissues such as the endometrium, it behaves as an agonist, hence tamoxifen may be characterized as a mixed agonist/antagonist. It has been the standard endocrine (anti-estrogen) therapy for hormone receptor-positive early breast cancer in pre-menopausal women, although aromatase inhibitors have been proposed.

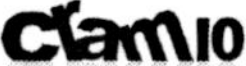





Go to **Cram101.com** for Interactive Practice Exams for this book or virtually any of your books.
And, **NEVER** highlight a book again!

| | |
|---|---|
| Aphasia | Aphasia meaning speechless, is an acquired language disorder in which there is an impairment of any language modality. This may include difficulty in producing or comprehending spoken or written language.<br><br>Traditionally, aphasia suggests the total impairment of language ability, and dysphasia a degree of impairment less than total. |
| Dementia | Dementia is a serious loss of cognitive ability in a previously unimpaired person, beyond what might be expected from normal aging. It may be static, the result of a unique global brain injury, or progressive, resulting in long-term decline due to damage or disease in the body. Although dementia is far more common in the geriatric population, it may occur in any stage of adulthood. |
| Jamais vu | In psychology, jamais vu is the phenomenon of experiencing a situation that one recognises but that nonetheless seems very unfamiliar.<br><br>Linguistics<br><br>From a linguistic perspective, the phenomenon that a word after frequent repetition seems to lose its meaning is connected with the very nature of words. A word as a unit of language has three characteristics:<br><br>• It has form, i.e. it is shaped out of sounds or, in the case of written language, out of letters (characters).<br>• It has function, which (among other things) means that it operates in a meaningful sentence.<br>• It has meaning, which implies that it refers to a certain unit of thought (a concept or an idea) within a context.<br><br>However, when a word is repeated over and over again, it is in fact only the form which is repeated. |

Go to **Cram101.com** for Interactive Practice Exams for this book or virtually any of your books.
And, **NEVER** highlight a book again!

| | |
|---|---|
| Ganser syndrome | Ganser syndrome is a rare dissociative disorder previously classified as a factitious disorder. It is characterized by nonsensical or wrong answers to questions or doing things incorrectly, other dissociative symptoms such as fugue, amnesia or conversion disorder, often with visual pseudohallucinations and a decreased state of consciousness. It is also sometimes called nonsense syndrome, balderdash syndrome, syndrome of approximate answers, pseudodementia, hysterical pseudodementia or prison psychosis. |
| Complex | A complex is a core pattern of emotions, memories, perceptions, and wishes in the personal unconscious organized around a common theme, such as power or status (Schultz, D. ' Schultz, S., 2009). Primarily a psychoanalytic term, it is found extensively in the works of Carl Jung and Sigmund Freud.<br><br>An example of a complex would be as follows: if you had a leg amputated when you were a child, this would influence your life in profound ways, even if you were wonderfully successful in overcoming the handicap. |
| Bender-Gestalt Test | The Bender Visual Motor Gestalt Test, or simply the Bender-Gestalt test, is a psychological test first developed by child neuropsychiatrist Lauretta Bender. The test is used to evaluate "visual-motor maturity", to screen for developmental disorders, or to assess neurological function or brain damage.<br><br>The original test consists of nine figures, each on its own 3 × 5 card. |
| Onset | Onset refers to the beginning of a musical note or other sound, in which the amplitude rises from zero to an initial peak. It is related to (but different from) the concept of a transient: all musical notes have an onset, but do not necessarily include an initial transient.<br><br>In phonetics the term is used differently - see syllable onset. |

Go to **Cram101.com** for Interactive Practice Exams for this book or virtually any of your books.
And, **NEVER** highlight a book again!

| | |
|---|---|
| Dyslexia | Dyslexia is a broad term defining a learning disability that impairs a person's fluency or accuracy in being able to read, speak, and spell. and which can manifest itself as a difficulty with phonological awareness, phonological decoding, orthographic coding, auditory short-term memory, and/or rapid naming. Dyslexia is separate and distinct from reading difficulties resulting from other causes, such as a non-neurological deficiency with vision or hearing, or from poor or inadequate reading instruction. |
| Slow-wave sleep | Slow-wave sleep often referred to as deep sleep, consists of stages 3 and 4 of non-rapid eye movement sleep, according to the Rechtschaffen ' Kales (R ' K) standard of 1968. As of 2008, the American Academy of Sleep Medicine (AASM) has discontinued the use of stage 4, such that the previous stages 3 and 4 now are combined as stage 3. An epoch (30 seconds of sleep) which consists of 20% or more slow wave (delta) sleep, now is considered to be stage 3.<br><br>The highest arousal thresholds (e.g. difficulty of awakening, such as by a sound of a particular volume) are observed in deep sleep. A person will typically feel more groggy when awoken from slow-wave sleep, and indeed, cognitive tests administered after awakening then indicate that mental performance is somewhat impaired for periods of up to 30 minutes or so, relative to awakenings from other stages. |
| Phobia | A phobia is an irrational, intense and persistent fear of certain situations, activities, things, animals, or people. The main symptom of this disorder is the excessive and unreasonable desire to avoid the feared stimulus. When the fear is beyond one's control, and if the fear is interfering with daily life, then a diagnosis under one of the anxiety disorders can be made. |
| Fear | Fear is a distressing emotion aroused by a perceived threat. It is a basic survival mechanism occurring in response to a specific stimulus, such as pain or the threat of danger. In short, fear is the ability to recognize danger and flee from it or confront it, also known as the Fight or Flight response. |
| Ictal | Ictal refers to a physiologic state or event such as a seizure, stroke or headache. The word originates from the Latin ictus, meaning a blow or a stroke. In electroencephalography (EEG), the recording during an actual seizure is said to be "ictal". |

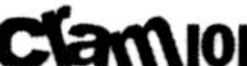





Go to **Cram101.com** for Interactive Practice Exams for this book or virtually any of your books.
And, **NEVER** highlight a book again!

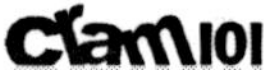



**Experience**

Experience as a general concept comprises knowledge of or skill in or observation of some thing or some event gained through involvement in or exposure to that thing or event. The history of the word experience aligns it closely with the concept of experiment.

The concept of experience generally refers to know-how or procedural knowledge, rather than propositional knowledge: on-the-job training rather than book-learning.

**Hallucination**

A hallucination, in the broadest sense of the word, is a perception in the absence of a stimulus. In a stricter sense, hallucinations are defined as perceptions in a conscious and awake state in the absence of external stimuli which have qualities of real perception, in that they are vivid, substantial, and located in external objective space. The latter definition distinguishes hallucinations from the related phenomena of dreaming, which does not involve wakefulness; illusion, which involves distorted or misinterpreted real perception; imagery, which does not mimic real perception and is under voluntary control; and pseudohallucination, which does not mimic real perception, but is not under voluntary control.

**Autosomal dominant nocturnal frontal lobe epilepsy**

Autosomal dominant nocturnal frontal lobe epilepsy is a rare epileptic disorder that causes frequent violent seizures during sleep. These seizures often involve complex motor movements, such as hand clenching, arm raising/lowering, and knee bending. Vocalizations such as shouting, moaning, or crying are also common.

**Amnesia**

Amnesia is a condition in which memory is disturbed or lost. The causes of amnesia have traditionally been divided into categories. Functional causes are psychological factors, such as mental disorder, post-traumatic stress or, in psychoanalytic terms, defense mechanisms.

**Transient epileptic amnesia**

Transient epileptic amnesia is a rare but probably underdiagnosed neurological condition which manifests as relatively brief and generally recurring episodes of amnesia caused by underlying temporal lobe epilepsy. Though descriptions of the condition are based on fewer than 100 cases published in the medical literature, and the largest single study to date included 50 people with Transient epileptic amnesia, Transient epileptic amnesia offers considerable theoretical significance as competing theories of human memory attempt to reconcile its implications.

Symptoms

Go to **Cram101.com** for Interactive Practice Exams for this book or virtually any of your books.
And, **NEVER** highlight a book again!

A person experiencing a Transient epileptic amnesia episode has very little short-term memory, so that there is profound difficulty remembering events in the past few minutes (anterograde amnesia), or of events in the hours prior to the onset of the attack, and even memories of important events in recent years may not be accessible during the amnestic event (retrograde amnesia).

**Atrophy**

Atrophy is the partial or complete wasting away of a part of the body. Causes of atrophy include mutations (which can destroy the gene to build up the organ), poor nourishment, poor circulation, loss of hormonal support, loss of nerve supply to the target organ, disuse or lack of exercise or disease intrinsic to the tissue itself. Hormonal and nerve inputs that maintain an organ or body part are referred to as trophic [noun] in medical practice. Trophic describes the trophic condition of tissue. A diminished muscular trophic is designated as atrophy.

**Tower of London Test**

The Tower of London test is a well-known test used in applied clinical neuropsychology for the assessment of executive functioning specifically to detect deficits in planning, which may occur due to a variety of medical and neuropsychiatric conditions. It is related to the classic problem-solving puzzle known as the Tower of Hanoi.

The test consists of two boards with pegs and several beads with different colors.

**Causality**

Causality is the relationship between an event (the cause) and a second event (the effect), where the second event is understood as a consequence of the first.

Though the causes and effects are typically related to changes or events, candidates include objects, processes, properties, variables, facts, and states of affairs; characterizing the causal relationship can be the subject of much debate.

**Disability**

A disability may be physical, cognitive, mental, sensory, emotional, developmental or some combination of these.
Disabilities is an umbrella term, covering impairments, activity limitations, and participation restrictions. An impairment is a problem in body function or structure; an activity limitation is a difficulty encountered by an individual in executing a task or action; while a participation restriction is a problem experienced by an individual in involvement in life situations.

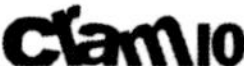





Go to **Cram101.com** for Interactive Practice Exams for this book or virtually any of your books.
And, **NEVER** highlight a book again!

| | |
|---|---|
| Anxiety | Anxiety is a psychological and physiological state characterized by somatic, emotional, cognitive, and behavioral components. The root meaning of the word anxiety is 'to vex or trouble'; in either the absence or presence of psychological stress, anxiety can create feelings of fear, worry, uneasiness and dread. Anxiety is considered to be a normal reaction to stress. |
| Differential diagnosis | A differential diagnosis is a systematic method used to identify unknowns. This method, essentially a process of elimination, is used by taxonomists to identify living organisms, and by physicians, nurse practitioners, physician assistants, and other trained medical professionals to diagnose the specific disease in a patient.<br><br>Not all medical diagnoses are differential ones: some diagnoses merely name a set of signs and symptoms that may have more than one possible cause, and some diagnoses are based on intuition or estimations of likelihood. In some cases, there will remain no diagnosis; this suggests the physician has made an error, or that the true diagnosis is unknown to medicine. Removing diagnoses from the list is done by making observations and using tests that should have different results, depending on which diagnosis is correct. |
| Panic | Panic is a sudden sensation of fear which is so strong as to dominate or prevent reason and logical thinking, replacing it with overwhelming feelings of anxiety and frantic agitation consistent with an animalistic fight or flight reaction. Panic may occur singularly in individuals or manifest suddenly in large groups as mass panic. The ancient Greeks credited the battle of Marathon's victory to Pan, using his name for the frenzied, frantic fear exhibited by the fleeing enemy soldiers. |
| Panic disorder | Panic disorder is an anxiety disorder characterized by recurring severe panic attacks. It may also include significant behavioral change lasting at least a month and of ongoing worry about the implications or concern about having other attacks. The latter are called anticipatory attacks (DSM-IVR). |
| Depression | Depression is a state of low mood and aversion to activity that can affect a person's thoughts, behaviour, feelings and physical well-being. It may include feelings of sadness, anxiety, emptiness, hopelessness, worthlessness, guilt, irritability, or restlessness. Depressed people may lose interest in activities that once were pleasurable, experience difficulty concentrating, remembering details, or making decisions, and may contemplate or attempt suicide. |
| Sexual dysfunction | Sexual dysfunction refers to a difficulty experienced by an individual or a couple during any stage of a normal sexual activity, including desire, arousal or orgasm. |

Go to **Cram101.com** for Interactive Practice Exams for this book or virtually any of your books.
And, **NEVER** highlight a book again!

To maximize the benefits of medications and behavioural techniques in the management of sexual dysfunction it is important to have a comprehensive approach to the problem,A thorough sexual history and assessment of general health and other sexual problems (if any) are very important. Assessing (performance) anxiety, guilt (associated with masturbation in many South-Asian men), stress and worry are integral to the optimal management of sexual dysfunction.

Psychosocial

Psychosocial refers to one's psychological development in and interaction with a social environment. The individual is not necessarily fully aware of this relationship with his or her environment. It was first commonly used by psychologist Erik Erikson in his stages of social development.

Medical error

Medical error is may be defined as a preventable adverse effect of care, whether or not it is evident or harmful to the patient. This might include an inaccurate or incomplete diagnosis or treatment of a disease, injury, syndromem behavior, infection, or other ailment. As a general acceptance, a medical error occurs when a health-care provider chose an inappropriate method of care or the health provider chose the right solution of care but executed it incorrectly. Medical errors are often described as human errors in healthcare.

Vasopressin

Vasopressin is a neurohypophysial hormone found in most mammals, including humans. Vasopressin is a peptide hormone that controls the reabsorption of molecules in the tubules of the kidneys by affecting the tissue's permeability. It also increases peripheral vascular resistance, which in turn increases arterial blood pressure. It plays a key role in homeostasis, and the regulation of water, glucose, and salts in the blood. It is derived from a preprohormone precursor that is synthesized in the hypothalamus and stored in vesicles at the posterior pituitary. Most of it is stored in the posterior pituitary to be released into the bloodstream; however, some AVP is also released directly into the brain, where it plays an important role in social behavior and bonding.

Cataplexy

Cataplexy is a sudden and transient episode of loss of muscle tone, often triggered by emotions. It is a rare disease (prevalence of fewer than 5 per 10,000 in the community), but frequently affects people who have narcolepsy, a disorder whose principal signs are EDS (Excessive Daytime Sleepiness), sleep attacks, sleep paralysis, hypnagogic hallucinations and disturbed night-time sleep. Cataplexy is sometimes confused with epilepsy, in which a series of flashes or other stimuli can cause superficially similar seizures.

Go to **Cram101.com** for Interactive Practice Exams for this book or virtually any of your books.
And, **NEVER** highlight a book again!

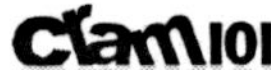



|  |  |
|---|---|
| Transient global amnesia | Transient global amnesia is "one of the most striking syndromes in clinical neurology" whose key defining characteristic is temporary but almost total disruption of short-term memory with a range of problems accessing older memories. A person in a state of Transient global amnesia exhibits no other signs of impaired cognitive functioning but recalls only the last few moments of consciousness plus deeply-encoded facts of the individual's past, such as his or her own name.<br><br>Symptoms<br><br>A person having an attack of Transient global amnesia has almost no capacity to establish new memories, but generally appears otherwise mentally alert and lucid, possessing full knowledge of self-identity and identity of close family, and maintaining intact perceptual skills and a wide repertoire of complex learned behavior. |
| Anticonvulsant | The anticonvulsants are a diverse group of pharmaceuticals used in the treatment of epileptic seizures. Anticonvulsants are also increasingly being used in the treatment of bipolar disorder, since many seem to act as mood stabilizers. The goal of an anticonvulsant is to suppress the rapid and excessive firing of neurons that start a seizure. Failing this, an effective anticonvulsant would prevent the spread of the seizure within the brain and offer protection against possible excitotoxic effects that may result in brain damage. |
| Carbamazepine | Carbamazepine is an anticonvulsant and mood stabilizing drug used primarily in the treatment of epilepsy and bipolar disorder, as well as trigeminal neuralgia. It is also used off-label for a variety of indications, including attention-deficit hyperactivity disorder (ADHD), schizophrenia, phantom limb syndrome, paroxysmal extreme pain disorder, neuromyotonia, intermittent explosive disorder, and post-traumatic stress disorder.<br><br>It has been seen as safe for pregnant women to use carbamazepine as a mood stabilizer. |

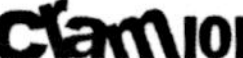





Go to **Cram101.com** for Interactive Practice Exams for this book or virtually any of your books.
And, **NEVER** highlight a book again!

| | |
|---|---|
| Drug interaction | A drug interaction is a situation in which a substance affects the activity of a drug, i.e. the effects are increased or decreased, or they produce a new effect that neither produces on its own. Typically, interaction between drugs come to mind (drug-drug interaction). However, interactions may also exist between drugs ' foods (drug-food interactions), as well as drugs ' herbs (drug-herb interactions). These may occur out of accidental misuse or due to lack of knowledge about the active ingredients involved in the relevant substances. |
| Interaction | Interaction is a kind of action that occurs as two or more objects have an effect upon one another. The idea of a two-way effect is essential in the concept of interaction, as opposed to a one-way causal effect. A closely related term is interconnectivity, which deals with the interactions of interactions within systems: combinations of many simple interactions can lead to surprising emergent phenomena. Interaction has different tailored meanings in various sciences. All systems are related and interdependent. Every action has a consequence. |
| Electroencephalography | Electroencephalography is the recording of electrical activity along the scalp produced by the firing of neurons within the brain. In clinical contexts, EEG refers to the recording of the brain's spontaneous electrical activity over a short period of time, usually 20-40 minutes, as recorded from multiple electrodes placed on the scalp. In neurology, the main diagnostic application of EE is in the case of epilepsy, as epileptic activity can create clear abnormalities on a standard EEG study. |
| Lamotrigine | Lamotrigine is an anticonvulsant drug used in the treatment of epilepsy and bipolar disorder. For epilepsy it is used to treat partial seizures, primary and secondary tonic-clonic seizures, and seizures associated with Lennox-Gastaut syndrome. Like many other anticonvulsant medications, Lamotrigine also seems to act as an effective mood stabilizer, and in fact has been the only U.S. Food and Drug Administration (FDA) approved drug for this purpose since lithium, a drug approved almost 30 years earlier. |
| Phenytoin | Phenytoin sodium is a commonly used antiepileptic. Phenytoin acts to suppress the abnormal brain activity seen in seizure by reducing electrical conductance among brain cells by stabilizing the inactive state of voltage-gated sodium channels. Aside from seizures, it is an option in the treatment of trigeminal neuralgia in the event that carbamazepine or other 1st line treatment is deemed inappropriate. |
| Barbiturate | Barbiturates are drugs that act as central nervous system depressants, and, by virtue of this, they produce a wide spectrum of effects, from mild sedation to total anesthesia. They are also effective as anxiolytics, as hypnotics, and as anticonvulsants. They have addiction potential, both physical and psychological. |

Go to **Cram101.com** for Interactive Practice Exams for this book or virtually any of your books.
And, **NEVER** highlight a book again!

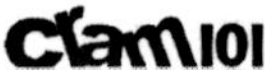



| | |
|---|---|
| Gabapentin | Gabapentin is a pharmaceutical drug, specifically a GABA analogue. It was originally developed for the treatment of epilepsy, and currently, gabapentin is widely used to relieve pain, especially neuropathic pain, as well as major depressive disorder.<br><br>Pharmacology<br><br>Gabapentin was initially synthesized to mimic the chemical structure of the neurotransmitter gamma-aminobutyric acid (GABA), but is not believed to act on the same brain receptors. |
| Pharmacotherapy | Pharmacotherapy is the treatment of disease through the administration of drugs. As such, it is considered part of the larger category of therapy.<br><br>Pharmacists are experts in pharmacotherapy and are responsible for ensuring the safe, appropriate, and economical use of medicines. As pharmacotherapy specialists, pharmacists have responsibility for direct patient care, often functioning as a member of a multidisciplinary team, and acting as the primary source of drug-related information for other healthcare professionals. |
| Phenobarbital | Phenobarbital or phenobarbitone (former BAN) is a barbiturate, first marketed as Luminal by Friedr. Bayer et comp. It is the most widely used anticonvulsant worldwide and the oldest still commonly used. |
| Topiramate | Topiramate is an anticonvulsant (antiepilepsy) drug. It was originally produced by Ortho-McNeil Neurologics and Noramco, Inc., both divisions of Johnson ' Johnson. It was discovered in 1979 by Bruce E. Maryanoff and Joseph F. Gardocki during their research work at McNeil Pharmaceutical. |
| Oxcarbazepine | Oxcarbazepine is an anticonvulsant and mood stabilizing drug, used primarily in the treatment of epilepsy. It is also used to treat anxiety and mood disorders, and benign motor tics. Oxcarbazepine is marketed as Trileptal by Novartis and available in some countries as a generic drug. |

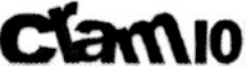





Go to **Cram101.com** for Interactive Practice Exams for this book or virtually any of your books.
And, **NEVER** highlight a book again!

| | |
|---|---|
| Pregabalin | Pregabalin is an anticonvulsant drug used for neuropathic pain and as an adjunct therapy for partial seizures with or without secondary generalization in adults. It has also been found effective for generalized anxiety disorder and is (as of 2007) approved for this use in the European Union. It was designed as a more potent successor to gabapentin. |
| Tiagabine | Tiagabine is an anti-convulsive medication produced by Cephalon and marketed under the brand name Gabitril. The drug was discovered at Novo Nordisk in Denmark in 1988 and was co-developed with Abbott. After a period of co-promotion, Cephalon licensed Tiagabine from Abbott/Novo and now is the exclusive producer. The medication is also used in the treatment of panic disorder, as are a few other anticonvulsants. |
| Biofeedback | Biofeedback is the process of becoming aware of various physiological functions using instruments that provide information on the activity of those same systems, with a goal of being able to manipulate them at will. Processes that can be controlled include brainwaves, muscle tone, skin conductance, heart rate and pain perception.<br><br>Biofeedback may be used to improve health or performance, and the physiological changes often occur in conjunction with changes to thoughts, emotions, and behavior. |
| Stimulation | Stimulation is the action of various agents (stimuli) on muscles, nerves, or a sensory end organ, by which activity is evoked; especially, the nervous impulse produced by various agents on nerves, or a sensory end organ, by which the part connected with the nerve is thrown into a state of activity.<br><br>The word is also often used metaphorically. For example, an interesting or fun activity can be described as "stimulating", regardless of its physical effects on nerves. |
| Lorazepam | Lorazepam is an high potency short to intermediate acting 3-hydroxy benzodiazepine drug which has all five intrinsic benzodiazepine effects: anxiolytic, amnesic, sedative/hypnotic, anticonvulsant and muscle relaxant. Lorazepam is used for the short-term treatment of anxiety, insomnia, acute seizures including status epilepticus and sedation of hospitalised patients, as well as sedation of aggressive patients. |

Go to **Cram101.com** for Interactive Practice Exams for this book or virtually any of your books.
And, **NEVER** highlight a book again!

| | |
|---|---|
| Antidepressant | An antidepressant is a psychiatric medication used to alleviate mood disorders, such as major depression and dysthymia and anxiety disorders such as social anxiety disorder. According to Gelder, Mayou '*Geddes (2005) people with a depressive illness will experience a therapeutic effect to their mood, however this will not be experienced in healthy individuals. Drugs including the monoamine oxidase inhibitors (MAOIs), tricyclic antidepressants (TCAs), tetracyclic antidepressants (TeCAs), selective serotonin reuptake inhibitors (SSRIs), and serotonin-norepinephrine reuptake inhibitors (SNRIs) are most commonly associated with the term. These medications are among those most commonly prescribed by psychiatrists and other physicians, and their effectiveness and adverse effects are the subject of many studies and competing claims. Many drugs produce an antidepressant effect, but restrictions on their use have caused controversy and off-label prescription a risk, despite claims of superior efficacy. |
| Antipsychotic | An antipsychotic is a tranquilizing psychiatric medication primarily used to manage psychosis (including delusions or hallucinations, as well as disordered thought), particularly in schizophrenia and bipolar disorder. A first generation of antipsychotics, known as typical antipsychotics, was discovered in the 1950s. Most of the drugs in the second generation, known as atypical antipsychotics, have been developed more recently, although the first atypical antipsychotic, clozapine, was discovered in the 1950s and introduced clinically in the 1970s. |

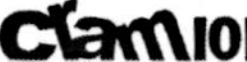





Go to **Cram101.com** for Interactive Practice Exams for this book or virtually any of your books.
And, **NEVER** highlight a book again!

| | |
|---|---|
| Epworth Sleepiness Scale | The Epworth Sleepiness Scale is a scale intended to measure daytime sleepiness that is measured by use of a very short questionnaire. This can be helpful in diagnosing sleep disorders. It was introduced in 1991 by Dr Murray Johns of Epworth Hospital in Melbourne, Australia. |
| Ethnic group | An ethnic group is a group of people whose members identify with each other, through a common heritage, often consisting of a common language, a common culture (often including a shared religion) and an ideology that stresses common ancestry or endogamy, "in general it is a highly biologically self-perpetuating group sharing an interest in a homeland connected with a specific geographical area, a common language and traditions, including food preferences, and a common religious faith". |
| Complex | A complex is a core pattern of emotions, memories, perceptions, and wishes in the personal unconscious organized around a common theme, such as power or status (Schultz, D. ' Schultz, S., 2009). Primarily a psychoanalytic term, it is found extensively in the works of Carl Jung and Sigmund Freud.<br><br>An example of a complex would be as follows: if you had a leg amputated when you were a child, this would influence your life in profound ways, even if you were wonderfully successful in overcoming the handicap. |
| Tower of London Test | The Tower of London test is a well-known test used in applied clinical neuropsychology for the assessment of executive functioning specifically to detect deficits in planning, which may occur due to a variety of medical and neuropsychiatric conditions. It is related to the classic problem-solving puzzle known as the Tower of Hanoi.<br><br>The test consists of two boards with pegs and several beads with different colors. |
| Neuropsychological Test | Neuropsychological tests are specifically designed tasks used to measure a psychological function known to be linked to a particular brain structure or pathway. They usually involve the systematic administration of clearly defined procedures in a formal environment. Neuropsychological tests are typically administered to a single person working with an examiner in a quiet office environment, free from distractions. |

Go to **Cram101.com** for Interactive Practice Exams for this book or virtually any of your books.
And, **NEVER** highlight a book again!

| | |
|---|---|
| Dementia | Dementia is a serious loss of cognitive ability in a previously unimpaired person, beyond what might be expected from normal aging. It may be static, the result of a unique global brain injury, or progressive, resulting in long-term decline due to damage or disease in the body. Although dementia is far more common in the geriatric population, it may occur in any stage of adulthood. |
| Polyneuropathy | Polyneuropathy is a neurological disorder that occurs when many peripheral nerves throughout the body malfunction simultaneously. It may be acute and appear without warning, or chronic and develop gradually over a longer period of time. Many polyneuropathies have both motor and sensory involvement; some also involve dysfunction of the autonomic nervous system. |
| Differential diagnosis | A differential diagnosis is a systematic method used to identify unknowns. This method, essentially a process of elimination, is used by taxonomists to identify living organisms, and by physicians, nurse practitioners, physician assistants, and other trained medical professionals to diagnose the specific disease in a patient.<br><br>Not all medical diagnoses are differential ones: some diagnoses merely name a set of signs and symptoms that may have more than one possible cause, and some diagnoses are based on intuition or estimations of likelihood. In some cases, there will remain no diagnosis; this suggests the physician has made an error, or that the true diagnosis is unknown to medicine. Removing diagnoses from the list is done by making observations and using tests that should have different results, depending on which diagnosis is correct. |
| Cognitive dysfunction | Cognitive dysfunction is defined as unusually poor mental function, associated with confusion, forgetfulness and difficulty concentrating. A number of medical or psychiatric conditions and treatments can cause such symptoms, including heavy metal poisoning (in particular mercury poisoning), menopause, fibromyalgia, ADHD and sleep disorders (including disrupted sleep). The term brain fog is not commonly used to describe people with dementia or other conditions that are known to cause confusion and memory problems, but it can be used as a synonym for sleep inertia or grogginess upon being awakened from deep sleep. |
| Fear | Fear is a distressing emotion aroused by a perceived threat. It is a basic survival mechanism occurring in response to a specific stimulus, such as pain or the threat of danger. In short, fear is the ability to recognize danger and flee from it or confront it, also known as the Fight or Flight response. |

Go to **Cram101.com** for Interactive Practice Exams for this book or virtually any of your books.
And, **NEVER** highlight a book again!

| | |
|---|---|
| Depression | Depression is a state of low mood and aversion to activity that can affect a person's thoughts, behaviour, feelings and physical well-being. It may include feelings of sadness, anxiety, emptiness, hopelessness, worthlessness, guilt, irritability, or restlessness. Depressed people may lose interest in activities that once were pleasurable, experience difficulty concentrating, remembering details, or making decisions, and may contemplate or attempt suicide. |
| Mania | Mania, the presence of which is a criterion for certain psychiatric diagnoses, is a state of abnormally elevated or irritable mood, arousal, and/or energy levels. In a sense, it is the opposite of depression.<br><br>In addition to mood disorders, individuals may exhibit manic behavior as a result of drug intoxication (notably stimulants such as cocaine or methamphetamine), medication side effects (notably steroids), or malignancy. |
| Anticonvulsant | The anticonvulsants are a diverse group of pharmaceuticals used in the treatment of epileptic seizures. Anticonvulsants are also increasingly being used in the treatment of bipolar disorder, since many seem to act as mood stabilizers. The goal of an anticonvulsant is to suppress the rapid and excessive firing of neurons that start a seizure. Failing this, an effective anticonvulsant would prevent the spread of the seizure within the brain and offer protection against possible excitotoxic effects that may result in brain damage. |
| Tabes dorsalis | Tabes dorsalis is a slow degeneration of the sensory neurons that carry information. The degenerating nerves are in the dorsal columns (posterior columns) of the spinal cord (the portion closest to the back of the body) and carry information that help maintain a person's sense of position (proprioception), vibration, and discriminative touch.<br><br>Cause<br><br>Tabes dorsalis is caused by demyelination secondary to an untreated syphilis infection. |

Go to **Cram101.com** for Interactive Practice Exams for this book or virtually any of your books.
And, **NEVER** highlight a book again!

| | |
|---|---|
| Delirium | Delirium is a common and severe neuropsychiatric syndrome with core features of acute onset and fluctuating course, attentional deficits and generalized severe disorganization of behavior. It typically involves other cognitive deficits, changes in arousal (hyperactive, hypoactive, or mixed), perceptual deficits, altered sleep-wake cycle, and psychotic features such as hallucinations and delusions. It is often caused by a disease process 'outside' the brain, such as common forms of infection (UTI, pneumonia) or by drug effects, particularly anticholinergic or other CNS depressants (benzodiazepines and opioids). |
| Delirium tremens | Delirium tremens is an acute episode of delirium that is usually caused by withdrawal from alcohol, first described in 1813. Benzodiazepines are the treatment of choice for delirium tremens.<br><br>Withdrawal from sedative-hypnotics other than alcohol, such as benzodiazepines or barbiturates can also result in seizures, Delirium tremens and death if not properly managed. Withdrawal from other drugs which are not sedative-hypnotics, such as opioids, marijuana, cocaine etc. |
| Aphasia | Aphasia meaning speechless, is an acquired language disorder in which there is an impairment of any language modality. This may include difficulty in producing or comprehending spoken or written language.<br><br>Traditionally, aphasia suggests the total impairment of language ability, and dysphasia a degree of impairment less than total. |
| Electroencephalography | Electroencephalography is the recording of electrical activity along the scalp produced by the firing of neurons within the brain. In clinical contexts, EEG refers to the recording of the brain's spontaneous electrical activity over a short period of time, usually 20-40 minutes, as recorded from multiple electrodes placed on the scalp. In neurology, the main diagnostic application of EE is in the case of epilepsy, as epileptic activity can create clear abnormalities on a standard EEG study. |

Go to **Cram101.com** for Interactive Practice Exams for this book or virtually any of your books.
And, **NEVER** highlight a book again!

|  |  |
| --- | --- |
| Relapse | A relapse occurs when a person is affected again by a condition that affected him in the past. This could be a medical or psychological condition such as depression, Facebook, an eating disorder, schizophrenia, bipolar disorder, multiple sclerosis, cancer or an addiction to a drug and or substance abuse.<br><br>For example, if someone who had problems with alcohol were to give up alcohol and then later start drinking again, this drinking might be considered a relapse. |
| Causality | Causality is the relationship between an event (the cause) and a second event (the effect), where the second event is understood as a consequence of the first.<br><br>Though the causes and effects are typically related to changes or events, candidates include objects, processes, properties, variables, facts, and states of affairs; characterizing the causal relationship can be the subject of much debate. |
| Herpes simplex | Herpes simplex is a viral disease caused by both herpes simplex virus type 1 (HSV-1) and type 2 (HSV-2). Infection with the herpes virus is categorized into one of several distinct disorders based on the site of infection. Oral herpes, the visible symptoms of which are colloquially called cold sores or fever blisters, infects the face and mouth. |
| Catatonia | Catatonia is a syndrome of psychological and motorological disturbances. It was first described in 1874: Die Katatonie oder das Spannungirresein (Catatonia or Tension Insanity).<br><br>In the current Diagnostic and Statistical Manual of Mental Disorders published by the American Psychiatric Association (DSM-IV) it is not recognized as a separate disorder, but is associated with psychiatric conditions such as schizophrenia (catatonic type), bipolar disorder, post-traumatic stress disorder, depression and other mental disorders, as well as drug abuse or overdose (or both). |
| Amnesia | Amnesia is a condition in which memory is disturbed or lost. The causes of amnesia have traditionally been divided into categories. Functional causes are psychological factors, such as mental disorder, post-traumatic stress or, in psychoanalytic terms, defense mechanisms. |

Chapter 7. Intracranial Infections,



Go to **Cram101.com** for Interactive Practice Exams for this book or virtually any of your books.
And, **NEVER** highlight a book again!

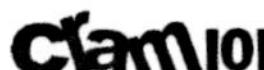



| | |
|---|---|
| Retrograde amnesia | Retrograde amnesia is a form of amnesia where someone is unable to recall events that occurred before the development of the amnesia. The term is used to categorise patterns of symptoms, rather than to indicate a particular cause or etiology; it is therefore a syndrome and not a disease.<br><br>Both retrograde amnesia and anterograde amnesia can occur together in the same patient. |

Go to **Cram101.com** for Interactive Practice Exams for this book or virtually any of your books.
And, **NEVER** highlight a book again!

| | |
|---|---|
| Causality | Causality is the relationship between an event (the cause) and a second event (the effect), where the second event is understood as a consequence of the first.<br><br>Though the causes and effects are typically related to changes or events, candidates include objects, processes, properties, variables, facts, and states of affairs; characterizing the causal relationship can be the subject of much debate. |
| Dementia | Dementia is a serious loss of cognitive ability in a previously unimpaired person, beyond what might be expected from normal aging. It may be static, the result of a unique global brain injury, or progressive, resulting in long-term decline due to damage or disease in the body. Although dementia is far more common in the geriatric population, it may occur in any stage of adulthood. |
| Aphasia | Aphasia meaning speechless, is an acquired language disorder in which there is an impairment of any language modality. This may include difficulty in producing or comprehending spoken or written language.<br><br>Traditionally, aphasia suggests the total impairment of language ability, and dysphasia a degree of impairment less than total. |
| Differential diagnosis | A differential diagnosis is a systematic method used to identify unknowns. This method, essentially a process of elimination, is used by taxonomists to identify living organisms, and by physicians, nurse practitioners, physician assistants, and other trained medical professionals to diagnose the specific disease in a patient.<br><br>Not all medical diagnoses are differential ones: some diagnoses merely name a set of signs and symptoms that may have more than one possible cause, and some diagnoses are based on intuition or estimations of likelihood. In some cases, there will remain no diagnosis; this suggests the physician has made an error, or that the true diagnosis is unknown to medicine. Removing diagnoses from the list is done by making observations and using tests that should have different results, depending on which diagnosis is correct. |

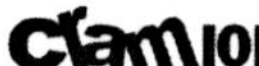





Go to **Cram101.com** for Interactive Practice Exams for this book or virtually any of your books.
And, **NEVER** highlight a book again!

|  |  |
|---|---|
| Anxiety | Anxiety is a psychological and physiological state characterized by somatic, emotional, cognitive, and behavioral components. The root meaning of the word anxiety is 'to vex or trouble'; in either the absence or presence of psychological stress, anxiety can create feelings of fear, worry, uneasiness and dread. Anxiety is considered to be a normal reaction to stress. |
| Depression | Depression is a state of low mood and aversion to activity that can affect a person's thoughts, behaviour, feelings and physical well-being. It may include feelings of sadness, anxiety, emptiness, hopelessness, worthlessness, guilt, irritability, or restlessness. Depressed people may lose interest in activities that once were pleasurable, experience difficulty concentrating, remembering details, or making decisions, and may contemplate or attempt suicide. |
| Hospital Anxiety and Depression Scale | Hospital Anxiety Depression Scale (Hospital Anxiety and Depression Scale) is commonly used by doctors to determine the levels of anxiety and depression that a patient is experiencing. It is a 10 point scale such that if a patient scores the lowest possible value of 1 they are considered to possibly need clinical psychiatric treatment. If the patient scores the maximum points (10) they will be considered clinically stable. |
| Electroencephalography | Electroencephalography is the recording of electrical activity along the scalp produced by the firing of neurons within the brain. In clinical contexts, EEG refers to the recording of the brain's spontaneous electrical activity over a short period of time, usually 20-40 minutes, as recorded from multiple electrodes placed on the scalp. In neurology, the main diagnostic application of EE is in the case of epilepsy, as epileptic activity can create clear abnormalities on a standard EEG study. |
| Substance abuse | Substance abuse, refers to a maladaptive pattern of use of a substance that is not considered dependent. The term "drug abuse" does not exclude dependency, but is otherwise used in a similar manner in nonmedical contexts. The terms have a huge range of definitions related to taking a psychoactive drug or performance enhancing drug for a non-therapeutic or non-medical effect. |
| Amnesia | Amnesia is a condition in which memory is disturbed or lost. The causes of amnesia have traditionally been divided into categories. Functional causes are psychological factors, such as mental disorder, post-traumatic stress or, in psychoanalytic terms, defense mechanisms. |
| Brain damage | Brain damage is the destruction or degeneration of brain cells. Brain injuries occur due to a wide range of internal and external factors. A common category with the greatest number of injuries is traumatic brain injury (TBI) following physical trauma or head injury from an outside source, and the term acquired brain injury (ABI) is used in appropriate circles, to differentiate brain injuries occurring after birth from injury due to a disorder or congenital malady. |

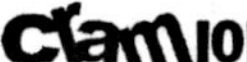





Go to **Cram101.com** for Interactive Practice Exams for this book or virtually any of your books.
And, **NEVER** highlight a book again!

Retinal

Retinal, is one of the many forms of vitamin A (the number of which varies from species to species). Retinal is a polyene chromophore, and bound to proteins called opsins, is the chemical basis of animal vision. Bound to proteins called type 1 rhodopsins, retinal allows certain microorganisms to convert light into metabolic energy.

Retinal migraine

Retinal migraine is a retinal disease often accompanied by migraine headache and typically affects only one eye. It is caused by a vascular spasm behind the affected eye.

Symptoms

Retinal migraine is associated with transient monocular visual loss (scotoma) in one eye lasting less than one hour.

Pathophysiology

Pathophysiology is the study of the changes of normal mechanical, physical, and biochemical functions, either caused by a disease, or resulting from an abnormal syndrome. More formally, it is the branch of medicine which deals with any disturbances of body functions, caused by disease or prodromal symptoms.

An alternative definition is "the study of the biological and physical manifestations of disease as they correlate with the underlying abnormalities and physiological disturbances."

The study of pathology and the study of pathophysiology often involves substantial overlap in diseases and processes, but pathology emphasizes direct observations, while pathophysiology emphasizes quantifiable measurements.

Neuroticism

Neuroticism is a fundamental personality trait in the study of psychology. It is an enduring tendency to experience negative emotional states. Individuals who score high on neuroticism are more likely than the average to experience such feelings as anxiety, anger, guilt, and depressed mood.

Go to **Cram101.com** for Interactive Practice Exams for this book or virtually any of your books.
And, **NEVER** highlight a book again!

Chronic

In medicine, a chronic disease is a disease that is long-lasting or recurrent. The term chronic describes the course of the disease, or its rate of onset and development. A chronic course is distinguished from a recurrent course; recurrent diseases relapse repeatedly, with periods of remission in between. As an adjective, chronic can refer to a persistent and lasting medical condition. Chronicity is usually applied to a condition that lasts more than three months. The opposite of chronic is acute.

Duality

In the context of a Community of practice the notion of a duality is used to capture the idea of the tension between two opposing forces which become a driving force for change and creativity. Wenger (Wenger 1998) uses the concept of dualities to examine the forces that create and sustain a Community of Practice. He describes a duality thus: '... a single conceptual unit that is formed by two inseparable and mutually constitutive elements whose inherent tensions and complementarity give the concept richness and dynamism' (Wenger 1998, p. 66).

Buspirone

Buspirone is a psychoactive drug and pharmaceutical medication of the piperazine and azapirone chemical classes. It is used primarily as an anxiolytic, specifically for generalized anxiety disorder. Bristol-Myers Squibb (BMS) gained Food and Drug Administration (FDA) approval for buspirone in 1986 for generalized anxiety disorder only, and it became available as a generic in 2001.

Psychosis

Psychosis means abnormal condition of the mind, and is a generic psychiatric term for a mental state often described as involving a "loss of contact with reality". People suffering from psychosis are described as psychotic. Psychosis is given to the more severe forms of psychiatric disorder, during which hallucinations and delusions and impaired insight may occur.

Hallucination

A hallucination, in the broadest sense of the word, is a perception in the absence of a stimulus. In a stricter sense, hallucinations are defined as perceptions in a conscious and awake state in the absence of external stimuli which have qualities of real perception, in that they are vivid, substantial, and located in external objective space. The latter definition distinguishes hallucinations from the related phenomena of dreaming, which does not involve wakefulness; illusion, which involves distorted or misinterpreted real perception; imagery, which does not mimic real perception and is under voluntary control; and pseudohallucination, which does not mimic real perception, but is not under voluntary control.

Illusion

An illusion is a distortion of the senses, revealing how the brain normally organizes and interprets sensory stimulation. While illusions distort reality, they are generally shared by most people. Illusions may occur with more of the human senses than vision, but visual illusions, optical illusions, are the most well known and understood.

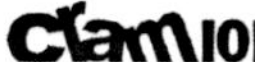





Go to **Cram101.com** for Interactive Practice Exams for this book or virtually any of your books.
And, **NEVER** highlight a book again!

| | |
|---|---|
| Cognitive dysfunction | Cognitive dysfunction is defined as unusually poor mental function, associated with confusion, forgetfulness and difficulty concentrating. A number of medical or psychiatric conditions and treatments can cause such symptoms, including heavy metal poisoning (in particular mercury poisoning), menopause, fibromyalgia, ADHD and sleep disorders (including disrupted sleep). The term brain fog is not commonly used to describe people with dementia or other conditions that are known to cause confusion and memory problems, but it can be used as a synonym for sleep inertia or grogginess upon being awakened from deep sleep. |

Go to **Cram101.com** for Interactive Practice Exams for this book or virtually any of your books.
And, **NEVER** highlight a book again!

|  |  |
| --- | --- |
| Dementia | Dementia is a serious loss of cognitive ability in a previously unimpaired person, beyond what might be expected from normal aging. It may be static, the result of a unique global brain injury, or progressive, resulting in long-term decline due to damage or disease in the body. Although dementia is far more common in the geriatric population, it may occur in any stage of adulthood. |
| Aphasia | Aphasia meaning speechless, is an acquired language disorder in which there is an impairment of any language modality. This may include difficulty in producing or comprehending spoken or written language.<br><br>Traditionally, aphasia suggests the total impairment of language ability, and dysphasia a degree of impairment less than total. |
| Apraxia | Apraxia is a disorder caused by damage to specific areas of the cerebrum, characterized by loss of the ability to execute or carry out learned purposeful movements, despite having the desire and the physical ability to perform the movements. It is a disorder of motor planning which may be acquired or developmental, but may not be caused by incoordination, sensory loss, or failure to comprehend simple commands (which can be tested by asking the person to recognize the correct movement from a series). Apraxia should not be confused with ataxia, a lack of coordination of movements, aphasia, an inability to produce and/or comprehend language; abulia, the lack of desire to carry out an action; or allochiria, in which patients perceive stimuli to one side of the body as occurring on the other. |
| Language disorder | Language disorders or language impairments are disorders that involve the processing of linguistic information. Problems that may be experienced can involve grammar (syntax and/or morphology), semantics (meaning), or other aspects of language. These problems may be receptive (involving impaired language comprehension), expressive (involving language production), or a combination of both. |
| Differential diagnosis | A differential diagnosis is a systematic method used to identify unknowns. This method, essentially a process of elimination, is used by taxonomists to identify living organisms, and by physicians, nurse practitioners, physician assistants, and other trained medical professionals to diagnose the specific disease in a patient. |

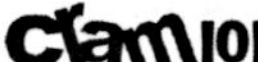





Go to **Cram101.com** for Interactive Practice Exams for this book or virtually any of your books.
And, **NEVER** highlight a book again!

Not all medical diagnoses are differential ones: some diagnoses merely name a set of signs and symptoms that may have more than one possible cause, and some diagnoses are based on intuition or estimations of likelihood. In some cases, there will remain no diagnosis; this suggests the physician has made an error, or that the true diagnosis is unknown to medicine. Removing diagnoses from the list is done by making observations and using tests that should have different results, depending on which diagnosis is correct.

| | |
|---|---|
| Mood disorder | Mood disorder is the term designating a group of diagnoses in the Diagnostic and Statistical Manual of Mental Disorders (DSM IV TR) classification system where a disturbance in the person's mood is hypothesized to be the main underlying feature. The classification is known as mood (affective) disorders in ICD 10.<br><br>English psychiatrist Henry Maudsley proposed an overarching category of affective disorder. |
| Neuroleptic malignant syndrome | Neuroleptic malignant syndrome is a life- threatening neurological disorder most often caused by an adverse reaction to neuroleptic or antipsychotic drugs. It generally presents with muscle rigidity, fever, autonomic instability and cognitive changes such as delirium, and is associated with elevated creatine phosphokinase (CPK). Incidence of the disease has declined since its discovery (due to changes in prescription habits), but it is still a potential danger to patients being treated with antipsychotics. |
| Psychosis | Psychosis means abnormal condition of the mind, and is a generic psychiatric term for a mental state often described as involving a "loss of contact with reality". People suffering from psychosis are described as psychotic. Psychosis is given to the more severe forms of psychiatric disorder, during which hallucinations and delusions and impaired insight may occur. |
| Neurofibrillary tangle | Neurofibrillary Tangles are aggregates of hyperphosphorylation tau that are most commonly known as a primary marker of Alzheimer's Disease. Their presence is also found in numerous other diseases known as Tauopathies. Little is known about their exact relationship to the different pathologies. |

Go to **Cram101.com** for Interactive Practice Exams for this book or virtually any of your books.
And, **NEVER** highlight a book again!

| | |
|---|---|
| Cerebral blood flow | Cerebral blood flow is the blood supply to the brain in a given time. In an adult, Cerebral blood flow is typically 750 millitres per minute or 15% of the cardiac output. This equates to 50 to 54 millilitres of blood per 100 grams of brain tissue per minute. Cerebral blood flow is tightly regulated to meet the brain's metabolic demands. Too much blood (a condition known as hyperemia) can raise intracranial pressure (ICP), which can compress and damage delicate brain tissue. Too little blood flow (ischemia) results if blood flow to the brain is below 18 to 20 ml per 100 g per minute, and tissue death occurs if flow dips below 8 to 10 ml per 100 g per minute. In brain tissue, a biochemical cascade known as the ischemic cascade is triggered when the tissue becomes ischemic, potentially resulting in damage to and death of brain cells. Medical professionals must take steps to maintain proper Cerebral blood flow in patients who have conditions like shock, stroke, and traumatic brain injury. |
| Metabolism | Metabolism is the set of chemical reactions that happen in living organisms to maintain life. These processes allow organisms to grow and reproduce, maintain their structures, and respond to their environments. Metabolism is usually divided into two categories. Catabolism breaks down organic matter, for example to harvest energy in cellular respiration. Anabolism uses energy to construct components of cells such as proteins and nucleic acids. |
| Blood alcohol content | Blood alcohol content, (also called Blood alcohol content, blood alcohol concentration, blood ethanol concentration, Blood Alcohol Level (BAL))is most commonly used as a metric of intoxication for legal or medical purposes. It is usually expressed as a fractional percentage in terms of volume of alcohol per liter of blood in the body. That is commonly expressed without units, or as a decimal with 2-3 significant digits followed by a percentage sign, which means 1/100 of the previous number (e.g., 0.0008 expressed as a percentage = 0.08%). |
| Kleine-Levin syndrome | Kleine-Levin Syndrome is a neurological disorder characterized by recurring periods of excessive amounts of sleep and altered behavior. At the onset of an episode the patient becomes drowsy and sleeps for most of the day and night (hypersomnolence), waking only to eat or go to the bathroom. When awake, the patient's whole demeanor is changed, often appearing "spacey" or childlike. |
| Hypersomnia | Hypersomnia is a disorder characterized by excessive amounts of sleepiness. There are two main categories of hypersomnia: primary hypersomnia and recurrent hypersomnia. Both have the same symptoms but differ in how often they occur. |

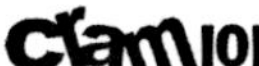





Go to **Cram101.com** for Interactive Practice Exams for this book or virtually any of your books.
And, **NEVER** highlight a book again!

| | |
|---|---|
| Hallucination | A hallucination, in the broadest sense of the word, is a perception in the absence of a stimulus. In a stricter sense, hallucinations are defined as perceptions in a conscious and awake state in the absence of external stimuli which have qualities of real perception, in that they are vivid, substantial, and located in external objective space. The latter definition distinguishes hallucinations from the related phenomena of dreaming, which does not involve wakefulness; illusion, which involves distorted or misinterpreted real perception; imagery, which does not mimic real perception and is under voluntary control; and pseudohallucination, which does not mimic real perception, but is not under voluntary control. |
| Illusion | An illusion is a distortion of the senses, revealing how the brain normally organizes and interprets sensory stimulation. While illusions distort reality, they are generally shared by most people. Illusions may occur with more of the human senses than vision, but visual illusions, optical illusions, are the most well known and understood. |
| Hypertension | Hypertension or high blood pressure is a cardiac chronic medical condition in which the systemic arterial blood pressure is elevated. It is the opposite of hypotension. Hypertension is classified as either primary (essential) or secondary. |
| Ganser syndrome | Ganser syndrome is a rare dissociative disorder previously classified as a factitious disorder. It is characterized by nonsensical or wrong answers to questions or doing things incorrectly, other dissociative symptoms such as fugue, amnesia or conversion disorder, often with visual pseudohallucinations and a decreased state of consciousness. It is also sometimes called nonsense syndrome, balderdash syndrome, syndrome of approximate answers, pseudodementia, hysterical pseudodementia or prison psychosis. |
| Multi-infarct dementia | Multi-infarct dementia, is one type of vascular dementia. Vascular dementia is the second most common form of dementia after Alzheimer's disease (AD) in older adults. Multi-infarct dementia is thought to be an irreversible form of dementia, and its onset is caused by a number of small strokes or sometimes, one large stroke. |
| Dementia with Lewy bodies | Dementia with Lewy bodies also known under a variety of other names including Lewy body dementia, diffuse Lewy body disease, cortical Lewy body disease, and senile dementia of Lewy type, is a type of dementia closely allied to both Alzheimers and Parkinson's Diseases. It is characterized anatomically by the presence of Lewy bodies, clumps of alpha-synuclein and ubiquitin protein in neurons, detectable in post-mortem brain biopsies.<br><br>Classification |

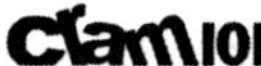





Go to **Cram101.com** for Interactive Practice Exams for this book or virtually any of your books.
And, **NEVER** highlight a book again!

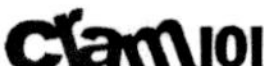



Dementia with Lewy bodies overlaps clinically with Alzheimer's disease and Parkinson's disease, but is more associated with the latter .

**Extrapyramidal symptoms**

The extrapyramidal system can be affected in a number of ways, which are revealed in a range of extrapyramidal symptoms also known as extrapyramidal side-effects (EPSE), such as akinesia (inability to initiate movement) and akathisia (inability to remain motionless).

Extrapyramidal symptoms are various movement disorders such as acute dystonic reactions, pseudoparkinsonism, or akathisia suffered as a result of taking dopamine antagonists, usually antipsychotic (neuroleptic) drugs, which are often used to control psychosis.

The Simpson-Angus Scale (SAS) and the Barnes Akathisia Rating Scale (BARS) are used to measure extrapyramidal symptoms.

**Frontotemporal dementia**

Frontotemporal dementia is a clinical syndrome caused by degeneration of the frontal lobe of the brain and may extend back to the temporal lobe. It is one of three syndromes caused by frontotemporal lobar degeneration, and the second most common early-onset dementia after Alzheimer's disease.

Signs and symptoms

Symptoms can be classified (roughly) into two groups which underlie the functions of the frontal lobe: behavioural symptoms (and/or personality change) and symptoms related to problems with executive function.

**Corticobasal degeneration**

Corticobasal degeneration or Corticobasal Ganglionic Degeneration (CBGD) is a rare progressive neurodegenerative disease involving the cerebral cortex and the basal ganglia. It is characterized by marked disorders in movement and cognitive dysfunction. Clinical diagnosis is difficult, as symptoms of CBD are often similar to those of other diseases, such as Parkinson's disease (PD) and progressive supranuclear palsy (PSP).

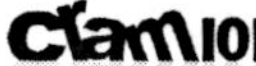





Go to **Cram101.com** for Interactive Practice Exams for this book or virtually any of your books.
And, **NEVER** highlight a book again!

| | |
|---|---|
| Progressive supranuclear palsy | Progressive supranuclear palsy (or the Steele-Richardson-Olszewski syndrome, after the Canadian physicians who described it in 1963) is a rare degenerative disease involving the gradual deterioration and death of selected areas of the brain.<br><br>Males and females are affected approximately equally and there is no racial, geographical or occupational predilection. Approximately 6 people per 100,000 population have Progressive supranuclear palsy.<br><br>It has been described as a tauopathy. |
| Herpes simplex | Herpes simplex is a viral disease caused by both herpes simplex virus type 1 (HSV-1) and type 2 (HSV-2). Infection with the herpes virus is categorized into one of several distinct disorders based on the site of infection. Oral herpes, the visible symptoms of which are colloquially called cold sores or fever blisters, infects the face and mouth. |
| Procedural memory | Procedural memory is our memory for how to do things. Procedural memory guides the processes we perform and most frequently resides below the level of conscious awareness. When needed, procedural memories are automatically retrieved and utilized for the execution of the integrated procedures involved in both cognitive and motor skills; from tying shoes to flying an airplane to reading. |
| Dopaminergic | Dopaminergic means related to the neurotransmitter dopamine. For example, certain proteins such as the dopamine transporter (DAT), vesicular monoamine transporter 2 ($VMAT_2$), and dopamine receptors can be classified as dopaminergic, and neurons which synthesize or contain dopamine and synapses with dopamine receptors in them may also be labeled as dopaminergic. Enzymes which regulate the biosynthesis or metabolism of dopamine such as aromatic L-amino acid decarboxylase (AAAD) or DOPA decarboxylase (DDC), monoamine oxidase (MAO), and catechol O-methyl transferase (COMT) may be referred to as dopaminergic as well. |
| Medical error | Medical error is may be defined as a preventable adverse effect of care, whether or not it is evident or harmful to the patient. This might include an inaccurate or incomplete diagnosis or treatment of a disease, injury, syndromem behavior, infection, or other ailment. As a general acceptance, a medical error occurs when a health-care provider chose an inappropriate method of care or the health provider chose the right solution of care but executed it incorrectly. Medical errors are often described as human errors in healthcare. |

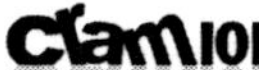





Go to **Cram101.com** for Interactive Practice Exams for this book or virtually any of your books.
And, **NEVER** highlight a book again!

| | |
|---|---|
| Fatal familial insomnia | Fatal familial insomnia is a very rare autosomal dominant inherited prion disease of the brain. It is almost always caused by a mutation to the protein $PrP^{C}$, but it can also develop spontaneously in patients without the inherited mutation in a variant called sporadic fatal insomnia (SFI). The mutated protein, called $PrP^{Sc}$, has been found in just 40 families worldwide, affecting about 100 people; if only one parent has the gene, the offspring have a 50% chance of inheriting it and developing the disease. |
| Stress | Stress is a term in psychology and biology, first coined in the biological context in the 1930s, which has in more recent decades become commonly used in popular parlance. It refers to the consequence of the failure of an organism - human or animal - to respond appropriately to emotional or physical threats, whether actual or imagined.<br><br>Signs of stress may be cognitive, emotional, physical or behavioral. |
| Amnesia | Amnesia is a condition in which memory is disturbed or lost. The causes of amnesia have traditionally been divided into categories. Functional causes are psychological factors, such as mental disorder, post-traumatic stress or, in psychoanalytic terms, defense mechanisms. |
| Gyrus | A gyrus is a ridge on the cerebral cortex. It is generally surrounded by one or more sulci (sl. sulcus). |
| Neurological examination | A neurological examination is the assessment of sensory neuron and motor responses, especially reflexes, to determine whether the nervous system is impaired. It can be used both as a screening tool and as an investigative tool, the former of which when examining the patient when there is no expected neurological deficit and the latter of which when examining a patient where you do expect to find abnormalities. If a problem is found either in an investigative or screening process then further tests can be carried out to focus on a particular aspect of the nervous system (such as lumbar punctures and blood tests). |
| Diogenes syndrome | Diogenes syndrome, is a disorder characterized by extreme self-neglect, domestic squalor, social withdrawal, apathy, compulsive hoarding of rubbish, and lack of shame. |

Go to **Cram101.com** for Interactive Practice Exams for this book or virtually any of your books.
And, **NEVER** highlight a book again!

The condition was first recognized in 1966 and designated Diogenes syndrome by Clark et al. Not only did he not hoard, but he actually sought human company by venturing daily to the Agora. Therefore, this eponym is considered to be a misnomer.

**Antidepressant**

An antidepressant is a psychiatric medication used to alleviate mood disorders, such as major depression and dysthymia and anxiety disorders such as social anxiety disorder. According to Gelder, Mayou '*Geddes (2005) people with a depressive illness will experience a therapeutic effect to their mood, however this will not be experienced in healthy individuals. Drugs including the monoamine oxidase inhibitors (MAOIs), tricyclic antidepressants (TCAs), tetracyclic antidepressants (TeCAs), selective serotonin reuptake inhibitors (SSRIs), and serotonin-norepinephrine reuptake inhibitors (SNRIs) are most commonly associated with the term. These medications are among those most commonly prescribed by psychiatrists and other physicians, and their effectiveness and adverse effects are the subject of many studies and competing claims. Many drugs produce an antidepressant effect, but restrictions on their use have caused controversy and off-label prescription a risk, despite claims of superior efficacy.

**Cognitive dysfunction**

Cognitive dysfunction is defined as unusually poor mental function, associated with confusion, forgetfulness and difficulty concentrating. A number of medical or psychiatric conditions and treatments can cause such symptoms, including heavy metal poisoning (in particular mercury poisoning), menopause, fibromyalgia, ADHD and sleep disorders (including disrupted sleep). The term brain fog is not commonly used to describe people with dementia or other conditions that are known to cause confusion and memory problems, but it can be used as a synonym for sleep inertia or grogginess upon being awakened from deep sleep.

**Community**

In biological terms, a community is a group of interacting organisms sharing a populated environment. In human communities, intent, belief, resources, preferences, needs, risks, and a number of other conditions may be present and common, affecting the identity of the participants and their degree of cohesiveness.

**Selective serotonin reuptake inhibitor**

Selective serotonin reuptake inhibitors or serotonin-specific reuptake inhibitor are a class of compounds typically used as antidepressants in the treatment of depression, anxiety disorders, and some personality disorders. They are also typically effective and used in treating some cases of insomnia.

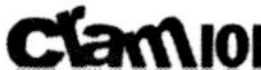





Go to **Cram101.com** for Interactive Practice Exams for this book or virtually any of your books.
And, **NEVER** highlight a book again!

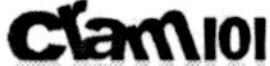



Selective serotonin reuptake inhibitors are believed to increase the extracellular level of the neurotransmitter serotonin by inhibiting its reuptake into the presynaptic cell, increasing the level of serotonin in the synaptic cleft available to bind to the postsynaptic receptor.

Cholinesterase

In biochemistry, cholinesterase is a family of enzymes that catalyze the hydrolysis of the neurotransmitter acetylcholine into choline and acetic acid, a reaction necessary to allow a cholinergic neuron to return to its resting state after activation.
There are two types:

- Acetylcholinesterase (EC 3.1.1.7) (AChE), also known as RBC cholinesterase, erythrocyte cholinesterase, or (most formally) acetylcholine acetylhydrolase, found primarily in the blood and neural synapses. Acetylcholinesterase exists in multiple molecular forms. In the mammalian brain the majority of AchE occurs as a tetrameric, G4 form (10) with much smaller amounts of a monomeric G1 (4S) form.

- Pseudocholinesterase (EC 3.1.1.8) (BChE or BuChE), also known as plasma cholinesterase, butyrylcholinesterase, or (most formally) acylcholine acylhydrolase, found primarily in the liver.

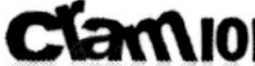





Go to **Cram101.com** for Interactive Practice Exams for this book or virtually any of your books.
And, **NEVER** highlight a book again!

| | |
|---|---|
| Depression | Depression is a state of low mood and aversion to activity that can affect a person's thoughts, behaviour, feelings and physical well-being. It may include feelings of sadness, anxiety, emptiness, hopelessness, worthlessness, guilt, irritability, or restlessness. Depressed people may lose interest in activities that once were pleasurable, experience difficulty concentrating, remembering details, or making decisions, and may contemplate or attempt suicide. |
| Brain damage | Brain damage is the destruction or degeneration of brain cells. Brain injuries occur due to a wide range of internal and external factors. A common category with the greatest number of injuries is traumatic brain injury (TBI) following physical trauma or head injury from an outside source, and the term acquired brain injury (ABI) is used in appropriate circles, to differentiate brain injuries occurring after birth from injury due to a disorder or congenital malady. |
| Hormone | A hormone is a chemical released by a cell or a gland in one part of the body that sends out messages that affect cells in other parts of the organism. Only a small amount of hormone is required to alter cell metabolism. In essence, it is a chemical messenger that transports a signal from one cell to another. All multicellular organisms produce hormones; plant hormones are also called phytohormones. Hormones in animals are often transported in the blood. Cells respond to a hormone when they express a specific receptor for that hormone. The hormone binds to the receptor protein, resulting in the activation of a signal transduction mechanism that ultimately leads to cell type-specific responses. |
| Stress | Stress is a term in psychology and biology, first coined in the biological context in the 1930s, which has in more recent decades become commonly used in popular parlance. It refers to the consequence of the failure of an organism - human or animal - to respond appropriately to emotional or physical threats, whether actual or imagined.<br><br>Signs of stress may be cognitive, emotional, physical or behavioral. |
| Polyneuropathy | Polyneuropathy is a neurological disorder that occurs when many peripheral nerves throughout the body malfunction simultaneously. It may be acute and appear without warning, or chronic and develop gradually over a longer period of time. Many polyneuropathies have both motor and sensory involvement; some also involve dysfunction of the autonomic nervous system. |

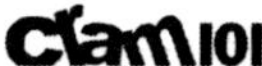





Go to **Cram101.com** for Interactive Practice Exams for this book or virtually any of your books.
And, **NEVER** highlight a book again!

| | |
|---|---|
| Dementia | Dementia is a serious loss of cognitive ability in a previously unimpaired person, beyond what might be expected from normal aging. It may be static, the result of a unique global brain injury, or progressive, resulting in long-term decline due to damage or disease in the body. Although dementia is far more common in the geriatric population, it may occur in any stage of adulthood. |
| Blood-brain barrier | The blood-brain barrier is a separation of circulating blood and the brain extracellular fluid (BECF) in the central nervous system (CNS). It occurs along all capillaries and consists of tight junctions around the capillaries that do not exist in normal circulation. Endothelial cells restrict the diffusion of microscopic objects (e.g. bacteria) and large or hydrophilic molecules into the cerebrospinal fluid (CSF), while allowing the diffusion of small hydrophobic molecules ($O_2$, hormones, $CO_2$). Cells of the barrier actively transport metabolic products such as glucose across the barrier with specific proteins. This barrier also includes a thick basement membrane and astrocytic endfeet. |
| Chronic | In medicine, a chronic disease is a disease that is long-lasting or recurrent. The term chronic describes the course of the disease, or its rate of onset and development. A chronic course is distinguished from a recurrent course; recurrent diseases relapse repeatedly, with periods of remission in between. As an adjective, chronic can refer to a persistent and lasting medical condition. Chronicity is usually applied to a condition that lasts more than three months. The opposite of chronic is acute. |
| Bipolar disorder | Bipolar disorder, also referred to as bipolar affective disorder or manic depression, is a psychiatric diagnosis that describes a category of mood disorders defined by the presence of one or more episodes of abnormally elevated energy levels, cognition, and mood with or without one or more depressive episodes. The elevated moods are clinically referred to as mania or, if milder, hypomania. Individuals who experience manic episodes also commonly experience depressive episodes, or symptoms, or mixed episodes in which features of both mania and depression are present at the same time. |
| Differential diagnosis | A differential diagnosis is a systematic method used to identify unknowns. This method, essentially a process of elimination, is used by taxonomists to identify living organisms, and by physicians, nurse practitioners, physician assistants, and other trained medical professionals to diagnose the specific disease in a patient. |

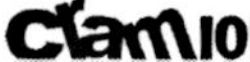





Go to **Cram101.com** for Interactive Practice Exams for this book or virtually any of your books.
And, **NEVER** highlight a book again!

Not all medical diagnoses are differential ones: some diagnoses merely name a set of signs and symptoms that may have more than one possible cause, and some diagnoses are based on intuition or estimations of likelihood. In some cases, there will remain no diagnosis; this suggests the physician has made an error, or that the true diagnosis is unknown to medicine. Removing diagnoses from the list is done by making observations and using tests that should have different results, depending on which diagnosis is correct.

Hypothyroidism

Hypothyroidism is a deficiency of thyroid hormone in humans and other vertebrates. Iodine deficiency is the most common cause of hypothyroidism worldwide but it can be caused by any number of other causes such as several conditions of the the thyroid gland, or less commonly, the pituitary gland or hypothalamus. It can result from a lack of a thyroid gland.

Schizophrenia

Schizophrenia is a mental disorder characterized by a disintegration of thought processes and of emotional responsiveness. It most commonly manifests as auditory hallucinations, paranoid or bizarre delusions, or disorganized speech and thinking, and it is accompanied by significant social or occupational dysfunction. The onset of symptoms typically occurs in young adulthood, with a global lifetime prevalence of about 0.3-0.7%.

Crisis

A crisis is any event that is, or expected to lead to, an unstable and dangerous situation affecting an individual, group, community or whole society. Crises are deemed to be negative changes in the security, economic, political, societal or environmental affairs, especially when they occur abruptly, with little or no warning. More loosely, it is a term meaning 'a testing time' or an 'emergency event'.

Causality

Causality is the relationship between an event (the cause) and a second event (the effect), where the second event is understood as a consequence of the first.

Though the causes and effects are typically related to changes or events, candidates include objects, processes, properties, variables, facts, and states of affairs; characterizing the causal relationship can be the subject of much debate.

Dystonia

Dystonia is a neurological movement disorder, in which sustained muscle contractions cause twisting and repetitive movements or abnormal postures. The disorder may be hereditary or caused by other factors such as birth-related or other physical trauma, infection, poisoning (e.g., lead poisoning) or reaction to pharmaceutical drugs, particularly neuroleptics. Treatment is difficult and has been limited to minimizing the symptoms of the disorder, since there is no cure available.

Go to **Cram101.com** for Interactive Practice Exams for this book or virtually any of your books.
And, **NEVER** highlight a book again!

| | |
|---|---|
| Antipsychotic | An antipsychotic is a tranquilizing psychiatric medication primarily used to manage psychosis (including delusions or hallucinations, as well as disordered thought), particularly in schizophrenia and bipolar disorder. A first generation of antipsychotics, known as typical antipsychotics, was discovered in the 1950s. Most of the drugs in the second generation, known as atypical antipsychotics, have been developed more recently, although the first atypical antipsychotic, clozapine, was discovered in the 1950s and introduced clinically in the 1970s. |
| Visual field | The term visual field is sometimes used as a synonym to field of view, though they do not designate the same thing. The visual field is the "spatial array of visual sensations available to observation in introspectionist psychological experiments", while 'field of view' "refers to the physical objects and light sources in the external world that impinge the retina". In other words, field of view is everything that (at a given time) causes light to fall onto the retina. |
| Vasopressin | Vasopressin is a neurohypophysial hormone found in most mammals, including humans. Vasopressin is a peptide hormone that controls the reabsorption of molecules in the tubules of the kidneys by affecting the tissue's permeability. It also increases peripheral vascular resistance, which in turn increases arterial blood pressure. It plays a key role in homeostasis, and the regulation of water, glucose, and salts in the blood. It is derived from a preprohormone precursor that is synthesized in the hypothalamus and stored in vesicles at the posterior pituitary. Most of it is stored in the posterior pituitary to be released into the bloodstream; however, some AVP is also released directly into the brain, where it plays an important role in social behavior and bonding. |
| Atrophy | Atrophy is the partial or complete wasting away of a part of the body. Causes of atrophy include mutations (which can destroy the gene to build up the organ), poor nourishment, poor circulation, loss of hormonal support, loss of nerve supply to the target organ, disuse or lack of exercise or disease intrinsic to the tissue itself. Hormonal and nerve inputs that maintain an organ or body part are referred to as trophic [noun] in medical practice. Trophic describes the trophic condition of tissue. A diminished muscular trophic is designated as atrophy. |
| Pyridoxine | Pyridoxine is one of the compounds that can be called vitamin $B_6$, along with pyridoxal and pyridoxamine. It differs from pyridoxamine by the substituent at the '4' position. It is often used as 'pyridoxine hydrochloride'.<br>Pyridoxine assists in the balancing of sodium and potassium as well as promoting red blood cell production. It is linked to cardiovascular health by decreasing the formation of homocysteine. Pyridoxine may help balance hormonal changes in women and aid the immune system. Lack of pyridoxine may cause anemia, nerve damage, seizures, skin problems, and sores in the mouth. |

Go to **Cram101.com** for Interactive Practice Exams for this book or virtually any of your books.
And, **NEVER** highlight a book again!

| | |
|---|---|
| Alcoholism | Alcoholism is a disabling addictive disorder. It is characterized by compulsive and uncontrolled consumption of alcohol despite its negative effects on the drinker's health, relationships, and social standing. Like other drug addictions, alcoholism is medically defined as a treatable disease. The term alcoholism is widely used, and was first coined in 1849 by Magnus Huss, but in medicine the term was replaced by the concepts of "alcohol abuse" and "alcohol dependence" in the 1980s DSM III. |
| Mood disorder | Mood disorder is the term designating a group of diagnoses in the Diagnostic and Statistical Manual of Mental Disorders (DSM IV TR) classification system where a disturbance in the person's mood is hypothesized to be the main underlying feature. The classification is known as mood (affective) disorders in ICD 10.<br><br>English psychiatrist Henry Maudsley proposed an overarching category of affective disorder. |
| Psychosis | Psychosis means abnormal condition of the mind, and is a generic psychiatric term for a mental state often described as involving a "loss of contact with reality". People suffering from psychosis are described as psychotic. Psychosis is given to the more severe forms of psychiatric disorder, during which hallucinations and delusions and impaired insight may occur. |
| Metabolism | Metabolism is the set of chemical reactions that happen in living organisms to maintain life. These processes allow organisms to grow and reproduce, maintain their structures, and respond to their environments. Metabolism is usually divided into two categories. Catabolism breaks down organic matter, for example to harvest energy in cellular respiration. Anabolism uses energy to construct components of cells such as proteins and nucleic acids. |
| Electroencephalography | Electroencephalography is the recording of electrical activity along the scalp produced by the firing of neurons within the brain. In clinical contexts, EEG refers to the recording of the brain's spontaneous electrical activity over a short period of time, usually 20-40 minutes, as recorded from multiple electrodes placed on the scalp. In neurology, the main diagnostic application of EE is in the case of epilepsy, as epileptic activity can create clear abnormalities on a standard EEG study. |

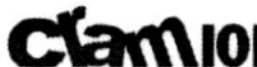





Go to **Cram101.com** for Interactive Practice Exams for this book or virtually any of your books.
And, **NEVER** highlight a book again!

|  |  |
|---|---|
| Selective serotonin reuptake inhibitor | Selective serotonin reuptake inhibitors or serotonin-specific reuptake inhibitor are a class of compounds typically used as antidepressants in the treatment of depression, anxiety disorders, and some personality disorders. They are also typically effective and used in treating some cases of insomnia.<br><br>Selective serotonin reuptake inhibitors are believed to increase the extracellular level of the neurotransmitter serotonin by inhibiting its reuptake into the presynaptic cell, increasing the level of serotonin in the synaptic cleft available to bind to the postsynaptic receptor. |
| Aphasia | Aphasia meaning speechless, is an acquired language disorder in which there is an impairment of any language modality. This may include difficulty in producing or comprehending spoken or written language.<br><br>Traditionally, aphasia suggests the total impairment of language ability, and dysphasia a degree of impairment less than total. |
| Epworth Sleepiness Scale | The Epworth Sleepiness Scale is a scale intended to measure daytime sleepiness that is measured by use of a very short questionnaire. This can be helpful in diagnosing sleep disorders. It was introduced in 1991 by Dr Murray Johns of Epworth Hospital in Melbourne, Australia. |
| Language disorder | Language disorders or language impairments are disorders that involve the processing of linguistic information. Problems that may be experienced can involve grammar (syntax and/or morphology), semantics (meaning), or other aspects of language. These problems may be receptive (involving impaired language comprehension), expressive (involving language production), or a combination of both. |

Go to **Cram101.com** for Interactive Practice Exams for this book or virtually any of your books.
And, **NEVER** highlight a book again!

| | |
|---|---|
| Dementia | Dementia is a serious loss of cognitive ability in a previously unimpaired person, beyond what might be expected from normal aging. It may be static, the result of a unique global brain injury, or progressive, resulting in long-term decline due to damage or disease in the body. Although dementia is far more common in the geriatric population, it may occur in any stage of adulthood. |
| Alcohol abuse | Alcohol abuse, as described in the DSM-IV, is a psychiatric diagnosis describing the recurring use of alcoholic beverages despite negative consequences. Alcohol abuse is sometimes referred to by the less specific term alcoholism. However, many definitions of alcoholism exist, and only some are compatible with alcohol abuse. |
| Blackout | A blackout is a phenomenon caused by the intake of alcohol or other substance in which long term memory creation is impaired or there is a complete inability to recall the past. Blackouts are frequently described as having effects similar to that of anterograde amnesia, in which the subject cannot create memories after the event that caused amnesia. 'Blacking out' is not to be confused with the mutually exclusive act of 'passing out', which means loss of consciousness. |
| Depressant | Depressants are psychoactive drugs that temporarily reduce the function or activity of a specific part of the body or brain. Examples of these kinds of effects may include anxiolysis, sedation, and hypotension. Due to their effects typically having a "down" quality to them, depressants are also occasionally referred to as "downers". |
| Abstinence | Abstinence is a voluntary restraint from indulging in bodily activities that are widely experienced as giving pleasure. Most frequently, the term refers to Sexual abstinence, or abstention from alcohol or food. The practice can arise from religious prohibitions or practical considerations. |
| Withdrawal | Withdrawal can refer to any sort of separation, but is most commonly used to describe the group of symptoms that occurs upon the abrupt discontinuation/separation or a decrease in dosage of the intake of medications, recreational drugs, and/or alcohol. In order to experience the symptoms of withdrawal, one must have first developed a physical dependence (often referred to as chemical dependency). This happens after consuming one or more of these substances for a certain period of time, which is both dose dependent and varies based upon the drug consumed. |
| Alcohol intoxication | Alcohol intoxication is a physiological state that occurs when a person has a high level of ethanol (alcohol) in their blood. Common symptoms of alcohol intoxication include slurred speech, euphoria, impaired balance, loss of muscle coordination (ataxia), flushed face, reddened eyes, reduced inhibition, and erratic behavior. In severe cases, it can cause coma or death. |

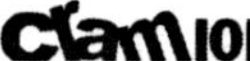





Go to **Cram101.com** for Interactive Practice Exams for this book or virtually any of your books.
And, **NEVER** highlight a book again!

| | |
|---|---|
| Delirium | Delirium is a common and severe neuropsychiatric syndrome with core features of acute onset and fluctuating course, attentional deficits and generalized severe disorganization of behavior. It typically involves other cognitive deficits, changes in arousal (hyperactive, hypoactive, or mixed), perceptual deficits, altered sleep-wake cycle, and psychotic features such as hallucinations and delusions. It is often caused by a disease process 'outside' the brain, such as common forms of infection (UTI, pneumonia) or by drug effects, particularly anticholinergic or other CNS depressants (benzodiazepines and opioids). |
| Delirium tremens | Delirium tremens is an acute episode of delirium that is usually caused by withdrawal from alcohol, first described in 1813. Benzodiazepines are the treatment of choice for delirium tremens.<br><br>Withdrawal from sedative-hypnotics other than alcohol, such as benzodiazepines or barbiturates can also result in seizures, Delirium tremens and death if not properly managed. Withdrawal from other drugs which are not sedative-hypnotics, such as opioids, marijuana, cocaine etc. |
| Alcoholic hallucinosis | Alcoholic hallucinosis is a complication of alcohol withdrawal in alcoholics. This develops about 12 to 24 hours after drinking stops and involves auditory hallucinations, most commonly accusatory or threatening voices. This condition is distinct from delirium tremens since it develops and resolves rapidly, involves a limited set of hallucinations and has no other physical symptoms. |
| Atrophy | Atrophy is the partial or complete wasting away of a part of the body. Causes of atrophy include mutations (which can destroy the gene to build up the organ), poor nourishment, poor circulation, loss of hormonal support, loss of nerve supply to the target organ, disuse or lack of exercise or disease intrinsic to the tissue itself. Hormonal and nerve inputs that maintain an organ or body part are referred to as trophic [noun] in medical practice. Trophic describes the trophic condition of tissue. A diminished muscular trophic is designated as atrophy. |
| Chlordiazepoxide | Chlordiazepoxide, is a sedative/hypnotic drug and benzodiazepine derivative. It is marketed under the trade names Klopoxid, Librax (also contains clidinium bromide), Libritabs, Librium, Mesural, Multum, Novapam, Risolid, Silibrin, Sonimen, Tropium, and Zetran. |

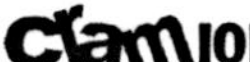





Go to **Cram101.com** for Interactive Practice Exams for this book or virtually any of your books.
And, **NEVER** highlight a book again!

| | |
|---|---|
| | Chlordiazepoxide was the first benzodiazepine to be synthesised and the discovery of chlordiazepoxide was by pure chance. |
| Cognitive dysfunction | Cognitive dysfunction is defined as unusually poor mental function, associated with confusion, forgetfulness and difficulty concentrating. A number of medical or psychiatric conditions and treatments can cause such symptoms, including heavy metal poisoning (in particular mercury poisoning), menopause, fibromyalgia, ADHD and sleep disorders (including disrupted sleep). The term brain fog is not commonly used to describe people with dementia or other conditions that are known to cause confusion and memory problems, but it can be used as a synonym for sleep inertia or grogginess upon being awakened from deep sleep. |
| Neuroleptic malignant syndrome | Neuroleptic malignant syndrome is a life- threatening neurological disorder most often caused by an adverse reaction to neuroleptic or antipsychotic drugs. It generally presents with muscle rigidity, fever, autonomic instability and cognitive changes such as delirium, and is associated with elevated creatine phosphokinase (CPK). Incidence of the disease has declined since its discovery (due to changes in prescription habits), but it is still a potential danger to patients being treated with antipsychotics. |
| Dendrite | Dendrites are the branched projections of a neuron that act to conduct the electrochemical stimulation received from other neural cells to the cell body, or soma, of the neuron from which the dendrites project. Electrical stimulation is transmitted onto dendrites by upstream neurons via synapses which are located at various points throughout the dendritic arbor. Dendrites play a critical role in integrating these synaptic inputs and in determining the extent to which action potentials are produced by the neuron. |
| Polyneuropathy | Polyneuropathy is a neurological disorder that occurs when many peripheral nerves throughout the body malfunction simultaneously. It may be acute and appear without warning, or chronic and develop gradually over a longer period of time. Many polyneuropathies have both motor and sensory involvement; some also involve dysfunction of the autonomic nervous system. |
| Metabolism | Metabolism is the set of chemical reactions that happen in living organisms to maintain life. These processes allow organisms to grow and reproduce, maintain their structures, and respond to their environments. Metabolism is usually divided into two categories. Catabolism breaks down organic matter, for example to harvest energy in cellular respiration. Anabolism uses energy to construct components of cells such as proteins and nucleic acids. |

Go to **Cram101.com** for Interactive Practice Exams for this book or virtually any of your books.
And, **NEVER** highlight a book again!

| | |
|---|---|
| Resistance | "Resistance" as initially used by Sigmund Freud, referred to patients blocking memories from conscious memory. This was a key concept, since the primary treatment method of Freud's talk therapy required making these memories available to the patient's consciousness.<br><br>"Resistance" expanded<br><br>Later, Freud described five different forms of resistance. |
| Medical error | Medical error is may be defined as a preventable adverse effect of care, whether or not it is evident or harmful to the patient. This might include an inaccurate or incomplete diagnosis or treatment of a disease, injury, syndromem behavior, infection, or other ailment. As a general acceptance, a medical error occurs when a health-care provider chose an inappropriate method of care or the health provider chose the right solution of care but executed it incorrectly. Medical errors are often described as human errors in healthcare. |
| Alcoholism | Alcoholism is a disabling addictive disorder. It is characterized by compulsive and uncontrolled consumption of alcohol despite its negative effects on the drinker's health, relationships, and social standing. Like other drug addictions, alcoholism is medically defined as a treatable disease. The term alcoholism is widely used, and was first coined in 1849 by Magnus Huss, but in medicine the term was replaced by the concepts of "alcohol abuse" and "alcohol dependence" in the 1980s DSM III. |
| Barbiturate | Barbiturates are drugs that act as central nervous system depressants, and, by virtue of this, they produce a wide spectrum of effects, from mild sedation to total anesthesia. They are also effective as anxiolytics, as hypnotics, and as anticonvulsants. They have addiction potential, both physical and psychological. |
| Bipolar disorder | Bipolar disorder, also referred to as bipolar affective disorder or manic depression, is a psychiatric diagnosis that describes a category of mood disorders defined by the presence of one or more episodes of abnormally elevated energy levels, cognition, and mood with or without one or more depressive episodes. The elevated moods are clinically referred to as mania or, if milder, hypomania. Individuals who experience manic episodes also commonly experience depressive episodes, or symptoms, or mixed episodes in which features of both mania and depression are present at the same time. |

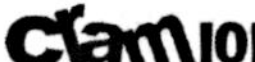





Go to **Cram101.com** for Interactive Practice Exams for this book or virtually any of your books.
And, **NEVER** highlight a book again!

## Chapter 11. Addictive and Toxic Disorders,

| | |
|---|---|
| Benton Visual Retention Test | The Benton Visual Retention Test is an individually administered test for ages 8-adult that measures visual perception and visual memory . It can also be used to help identify possible learning disabilities. The child is shown 10 designs, one at a time, and asked to reproduce each one as exactly as possible on plain paper from memory. |
| Benzodiazepine | A benzodiazepine is a psychoactive drug whose core chemical structure is the fusion of a benzene ring and a diazepine ring. The first benzodiazepine, chlordiazepoxide (Librium), was discovered accidentally by Leo Sternbach in 1955, and made available in 1960 by Hoffmann-La Roche, which has also marketed diazepam (Valium) since 1963. |
| Drug overdose | The term drug overdose describes the ingestion or application of a drug or other substance in quantities that are excessive. An overdose is widely considered harmful and dangerous as it can result in death. |
| Heroin | Heroin (diacetylmorphine (INN)), also known as diamorphine (BAN), is a semi-synthetic opioid drug synthesized from morphine, a derivative of the opium poppy. It is the 3,6-diacetyl ester of morphine (di (two)-acetyl-morphine). The white crystalline form is commonly the hydrochloride salt diacetylmorphine hydrochloride, though often adulterated thus dulling the sheen and consistency from that to a matte white powder, which diacetylmorphine freebase typically is. 90% of diacetylmorphine is thought to be produced in Afghanistan. |
| Opiate | In medicine, the term opiate describes any of the narcotic opioid alkaloids found as natural products in the opium poppy plant, as well as many semisynthetic chemical derivatives of such alkaloids.<br><br>Overview<br><br>Opiates are so named because they are constituents or derivatives of constituents found in opium, which is processed from the latex sap of the opium poppy, Papaver somniferum. The major biologically active opiates found in opium are morphine, codeine, papaverine and to a lesser extend thebaine, which is not narcotic. |
| Opioid | An opioid is a chemical that works by binding to opioid receptors, which are found principally in the central and peripheral nervous system and the gastrointestinal tract. The receptors in these organ systems mediate both the beneficial effects and the side effects of opioids. |

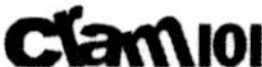





Go to **Cram101.com** for Interactive Practice Exams for this book or virtually any of your books.
And, **NEVER** highlight a book again!

Opioids are among the world's oldest known drugs; the use of the opium poppy for its therapeutic benefits predates recorded history.

Sedative

A sedative is a substance that induces sedation by reducing irritability or excitement.

At higher doses it may result in slurred speech, staggering gait, poor judgment, and slow, uncertain reflexes. Doses of sedatives such as benzodiazepines when used as a hypnotic to induce sleep tend to be higher than those used to relieve anxiety whereas only low doses are needed to provide calming sedative effects.

Neuropsychological Test

Neuropsychological tests are specifically designed tasks used to measure a psychological function known to be linked to a particular brain structure or pathway. They usually involve the systematic administration of clearly defined procedures in a formal environment. Neuropsychological tests are typically administered to a single person working with an examiner in a quiet office environment, free from distractions.

Cannabis

Cannabis is a genus of flowering plants that includes three putative species, Cannabis sativa, Cannabis indica, and Cannabis ruderalis. These three taxa are indigenous to Central Asia, and South Asia. Cannabis has long been used for fibre (hemp), for seed and seed oils, for medicinal purposes, and as a recreational drug.

Naloxone

Naloxone is a drug used to counter the effects of opiate overdose, for example heroin or morphine overdose. Naloxone is specifically used to counteract life-threatening depression of the central nervous system and respiratory system. Naloxone is also experimentally used in the treatment for congenital insensitivity to pain with anhidrosis (CIPA), an extremely rare disorder (1 in 125 million) that renders one unable to feel pain.

Amphetamine

Amphetamine or amfetamine (INN) is a psychostimulant drug of the phenethylamine class that is known to produce increased wakefulness and focus in association with decreased fatigue and appetite.

Brand names of medications that contain, or metabolize into, amphetamine include Adderall, Dexedrine, Dextrostat, Desoxyn, ProCentra, and Vyvanse, as well as Benzedrine in the past.

Go to **Cram101.com** for Interactive Practice Exams for this book or virtually any of your books.
And, **NEVER** highlight a book again!

| | |
|---|---|
| | The drug is also used recreationally and as a performance enhancer. |
| Methamphetamine | Methamphetamine, methylamphetamine, N-methylamphetamine, desoxyephedrine, and colloquially as "meth" or "crystal meth", is a psychostimulant of the phenethylamine and amphetamine class of drugs. It increases alertness, concentration, energy, and in high doses, can induce euphoria, enhance self-esteem, and increase libido. Methamphetamine has high potential for abuse and addiction by activating the psychological reward system via triggering a cascading release of dopamine, norepinephrine and serotonin in the brain. |
| Kleine-Levin syndrome | Kleine-Levin Syndrome is a neurological disorder characterized by recurring periods of excessive amounts of sleep and altered behavior. At the onset of an episode the patient becomes drowsy and sleeps for most of the day and night (hypersomnolence), waking only to eat or go to the bathroom. When awake, the patient's whole demeanor is changed, often appearing "spacey" or childlike. |
| Cocaine | Cocaine benzoylmethylecgonine (INN) is a crystalline tropane alkaloid that is obtained from the leaves of the coca plant. The name comes from "coca" in addition to the alkaloid suffix -ine, forming cocaine. It is a stimulant of the central nervous system, an appetite suppressant, and a topical anesthetic. |
| Hypersomnia | Hypersomnia is a disorder characterized by excessive amounts of sleepiness. There are two main categories of hypersomnia: primary hypersomnia and recurrent hypersomnia. Both have the same symptoms but differ in how often they occur. |
| Psychosis | Psychosis means abnormal condition of the mind, and is a generic psychiatric term for a mental state often described as involving a "loss of contact with reality". People suffering from psychosis are described as psychotic. Psychosis is given to the more severe forms of psychiatric disorder, during which hallucinations and delusions and impaired insight may occur. |
| Diazepam | Diazepam, first marketed as Valium by Hoffmann-La Roche, is a benzodiazepine derivative drug. Diazepam is also marketed in Australia as Antenex. It is commonly used for treating anxiety, insomnia, seizures including status epilepticus, muscle spasms, restless legs syndrome, alcohol withdrawal, benzodiazepine withdrawal and Ménière's disease. It may also be used before certain medical procedures (such as endoscopies) to reduce tension and anxiety, and in some surgical procedures to induce amnesia. It possesses anxiolytic, anticonvulsant, hypnotic, sedative, skeletal muscle relaxant, and amnestic properties. |

Go to **Cram101.com** for Interactive Practice Exams for this book or virtually any of your books.
And, **NEVER** highlight a book again!

| | |
|---|---|
| Ecstasy | Ecstasy is a subjective experience of total involvement of the subject, with an object of his or her awareness. Because total involvement with an object of our interest is not our ordinary experience since we are ordinarily aware also of other objects, the ecstasy is an example of altered state of consciousness characterized by diminished awareness of other objects or total lack of the awareness of surroundings and everything around the object. For instance, if one is concentrating on a physical task, then one might cease to be aware of any intellectual thoughts. |
| Propranolol | Propranolol is a non-selective beta blocker mainly used in the treatment of hypertension. It was the first successful beta blocker developed. Propranolol is available in generic form as propranolol hydrochloride, as well as an AstraZeneca and Wyeth product under the trade names Inderal, Inderal LA, Avlocardyl , Deralin, Dociton, Inderalici, InnoPran XL, Sumial, Anaprilinum (depending on marketplace and release rate), Bedranol SR (Sandoz). |
| Differential diagnosis | A differential diagnosis is a systematic method used to identify unknowns. This method, essentially a process of elimination, is used by taxonomists to identify living organisms, and by physicians, nurse practitioners, physician assistants, and other trained medical professionals to diagnose the specific disease in a patient.<br><br>Not all medical diagnoses are differential ones: some diagnoses merely name a set of signs and symptoms that may have more than one possible cause, and some diagnoses are based on intuition or estimations of likelihood. In some cases, there will remain no diagnosis; this suggests the physician has made an error, or that the true diagnosis is unknown to medicine. Removing diagnoses from the list is done by making observations and using tests that should have different results, depending on which diagnosis is correct. |
| Mescaline | Mescaline or 3,4,5-trimethoxyphenethylamine is a naturally-occurring psychedelic alkaloid of the phenethylamine class used mainly as an entheogen.<br><br>It occurs naturally in the peyote cactus (Lophophora williamsii), the San Pedro cactus (Echinopsis pachanoi) and the Peruvian Torch cactus (Echinopsis peruviana), and in a number of other members of the Cactaceae plant family. It is also found in small amounts in certain members of the Fabaceae (bean) family, including Acacia berlandieri. |

Go to **Cram101.com** for Interactive Practice Exams for this book or virtually any of your books.
And, **NEVER** highlight a book again!

| | |
|---|---|
| Phencyclidine | Phencyclidine (a complex clip of the chemical name 1-(1-phenylcyclohexyl)piperidine, commonly initialized as PCP), also known as angel dust and myriad other street names, is a recreational, dissociative drug formerly used as an anesthetic agent, exhibiting hallucinogenic and neurotoxic effects.<br><br>Developed in 1926, it was first patented in 1952 by the Parke-Davis pharmaceutical company and marketed under the brand name Sernyl. In chemical structure, PCP is an arylcyclohexylamine derivative, and, in pharmacology, it is a member of the family of dissociative anesthetics. |
| Alkyl nitrites | Alkyl nitrites are a group of chemical compounds based upon the molecular structure R-ONO. Formally they are alkyl esters of nitrous acid. They are distinct from nitro compounds ($R-NO_2$).<br><br>The first few members of the series are volatile liquids; methyl nitrite and ethyl nitrite are gaseous at room temperature and pressure. |
| Hallucination | A hallucination, in the broadest sense of the word, is a perception in the absence of a stimulus. In a stricter sense, hallucinations are defined as perceptions in a conscious and awake state in the absence of external stimuli which have qualities of real perception, in that they are vivid, substantial, and located in external objective space. The latter definition distinguishes hallucinations from the related phenomena of dreaming, which does not involve wakefulness; illusion, which involves distorted or misinterpreted real perception; imagery, which does not mimic real perception and is under voluntary control; and pseudohallucination, which does not mimic real perception, but is not under voluntary control. |
| Hallucinogen persisting perception disorder | Hallucinogen persisting perception disorder are reminiscent of those generated by the ingestion of hallucinogenic substances. Previous use of hallucinogens by the person is needed, though not sufficient, for diagnosing someone with the disorder. For an individual to be diagnosed with Hallucinogen persisting perception disorder, the symptoms cannot be due to another medical condition. |
| Nitrous oxide | Nitrous oxide, commonly known as laughing gas or sweet air, is a chemical compound with the formula $N_2O$. It is an oxide of nitrogen. At room temperature, it is a colorless non-flammable gas, with a slightly sweet odor and taste. |

Go to **Cram101.com** for Interactive Practice Exams for this book or virtually any of your books.
And, **NEVER** highlight a book again!

| | |
|---|---|
| Perception | In philosophy, psychology, and cognitive science, perception is the process of attaining awareness or understanding of sensory information. The word "perception" comes from the Latin words perceptio, percipio, and means "receiving, collecting, action of taking possession, apprehension with the mind or senses."<br><br>Perception is one of the oldest fields in psychology. The oldest quantitative law in psychology is the Weber-Fechner law, which quantifies the relationship between the intensity of physical stimuli and their perceptual effects. |
| Sodium valproate | Sodium valproate or valproate sodium (USAN) is the sodium salt of valproic acid and is an anticonvulsant used in the treatment of epilepsy and bipolar disorder, as well as other psychiatric conditions requiring the administration of a mood stabilizer. Sodium valproate can be used to control acute episodes of mania. Side effects can include tiredness, tremors, nausea, vomiting and sedation. |
| Vocation | A vocation is a term for an occupation to which a person is specially drawn or for which they are suited, trained or qualified. Though now often used in secular contexts, the meanings of the term originated in Christianity. |
| Tower of London Test | The Tower of London test is a well-known test used in applied clinical neuropsychology for the assessment of executive functioning specifically to detect deficits in planning, which may occur due to a variety of medical and neuropsychiatric conditions. It is related to the classic problem-solving puzzle known as the Tower of Hanoi.<br><br>The test consists of two boards with pegs and several beads with different colors. |
| Electroencephalography | Electroencephalography is the recording of electrical activity along the scalp produced by the firing of neurons within the brain. In clinical contexts, EEG refers to the recording of the brain's spontaneous electrical activity over a short period of time, usually 20-40 minutes, as recorded from multiple electrodes placed on the scalp. In neurology, the main diagnostic application of EE is in the case of epilepsy, as epileptic activity can create clear abnormalities on a standard EEG study. |

Go to **Cram101.com** for Interactive Practice Exams for this book or virtually any of your books.
And, **NEVER** highlight a book again!

| | |
|---|---|
| Haloperidol | Haloperidol is a typical antipsychotic. It is in the butyrophenone class of antipsychotic medications and has pharmacological effects similar to the phenothiazines.<br><br>Haloperidol is an older antipsychotic used in the treatment of schizophrenia and, more acutely, in the treatment of acute psychotic states and delirium. A long-acting decanoate ester is used as a long-acting injection given every 4 weeks to people with schizophrenia or related illnesses who have a poor compliance with medication and suffer frequent relapses of illness, or to overcome the drawbacks inherent to its orally administered counterpart that burst dosage increases risk or intensity of side effects. In some countries this can be involuntary under Community Treatment Orders. |
| Catatonia | Catatonia is a syndrome of psychological and motorological disturbances. It was first described in 1874: Die Katatonie oder das Spannungirresein (Catatonia or Tension Insanity).<br><br>In the current Diagnostic and Statistical Manual of Mental Disorders published by the American Psychiatric Association (DSM-IV) it is not recognized as a separate disorder, but is associated with psychiatric conditions such as schizophrenia (catatonic type), bipolar disorder, post-traumatic stress disorder, depression and other mental disorders, as well as drug abuse or overdose (or both). |
| Dopamine | Dopamine is a catecholamine neurotransmitter present in a wide variety of animals, including both vertebrates and invertebrates. In the brain, this substituted phenethylamine functions as a neurotransmitter, activating the five known types of dopamine receptors--$D_1$, $D_2$, $D_3$, $D_4$, and $D_5$--and their variants. Dopamine is produced in several areas of the brain, including the substantia nigra and the ventral tegmental area. |
| Epworth Sleepiness Scale | The Epworth Sleepiness Scale is a scale intended to measure daytime sleepiness that is measured by use of a very short questionnaire. This can be helpful in diagnosing sleep disorders. It was introduced in 1991 by Dr Murray Johns of Epworth Hospital in Melbourne, Australia. |
| Analgesic | An analgesic is any member of the group of drugs used to relieve pain (achieve analgesia). |

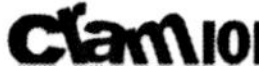





Go to **Cram101.com** for Interactive Practice Exams for this book or virtually any of your books.
And, **NEVER** highlight a book again!

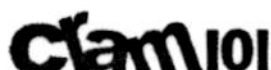



Analgesic drugs act in various ways on the peripheral and central nervous systems; they include paracetamol (para-acetylaminophenol, also known in the US as acetaminophen), the non-steroidal anti-inflammatory drugs (NSAIDs) such as the salicylates, and opioid drugs such as morphine and opium. They are distinct from anesthetics, which reversibly eliminate sensation.

Ethchlorvynol

Ethchlorvynol is a sedative and hypnotic medication. It has been used to treat insomnia, but has been largely superseded and is only offered where an intolerance or allergy to other drugs exists.

Along with expected sedative effects of relaxation and drowsiness, ethchlorvynol can cause skin rashes, faintness, restlessness and euphoria.

Glutethimide

Glutethimide is a hypnotic sedative that was introduced in 1954 as a safe alternative to barbiturates to treat insomnia. Before long, however, it had become clear that glutethimide was just as likely to cause addiction and caused similarly severe withdrawal symptoms. Doriden is the brand-name version of the drug; both the generic and brand-name forms are rarely prescribed today.

Progressive supranuclear palsy

Progressive supranuclear palsy (or the Steele-Richardson-Olszewski syndrome, after the Canadian physicians who described it in 1963) is a rare degenerative disease involving the gradual deterioration and death of selected areas of the brain.

Males and females are affected approximately equally and there is no racial, geographical or occupational predilection. Approximately 6 people per 100,000 population have Progressive supranuclear palsy.

It has been described as a tauopathy.

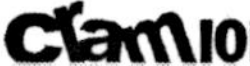





Go to **Cram101.com** for Interactive Practice Exams for this book or virtually any of your books.
And, **NEVER** highlight a book again!

| | |
|---|---|
| Complex | A complex is a core pattern of emotions, memories, perceptions, and wishes in the personal unconscious organized around a common theme, such as power or status (Schultz, D. ' Schultz, S., 2009). Primarily a psychoanalytic term, it is found extensively in the works of Carl Jung and Sigmund Freud. |
| | An example of a complex would be as follows: if you had a leg amputated when you were a child, this would influence your life in profound ways, even if you were wonderfully successful in overcoming the handicap. |

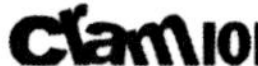





Go to **Cram101.com** for Interactive Practice Exams for this book or virtually any of your books.
And, **NEVER** highlight a book again!

|  |  |
| --- | --- |
| Dystonia | Dystonia is a neurological movement disorder, in which sustained muscle contractions cause twisting and repetitive movements or abnormal postures. The disorder may be hereditary or caused by other factors such as birth-related or other physical trauma, infection, poisoning (e.g., lead poisoning) or reaction to pharmaceutical drugs, particularly neuroleptics. Treatment is difficult and has been limited to minimizing the symptoms of the disorder, since there is no cure available. |
| Tardive dyskinesia | Tardive dyskinesia is a difficult-to-treat form of dyskinesia (disorder resulting in involuntary, repetitive body movements) that can be tardive (having a slow or belated onset). It frequently appears after long-term or high-dose use of antipsychotic drugs, or in children and infants as a side effect from usage of drugs for gastrointestinal disorders prevention.<br><br>Features<br><br>Tardive dyskinesia is characterized by repetitive, involuntary, purposeless movements, such as grimacing, tongue protrusion, lip smacking, puckering and pursing of the lips, and rapid eye blinking. |
| Differential diagnosis | A differential diagnosis is a systematic method used to identify unknowns. This method, essentially a process of elimination, is used by taxonomists to identify living organisms, and by physicians, nurse practitioners, physician assistants, and other trained medical professionals to diagnose the specific disease in a patient.<br><br>Not all medical diagnoses are differential ones: some diagnoses merely name a set of signs and symptoms that may have more than one possible cause, and some diagnoses are based on intuition or estimations of likelihood. In some cases, there will remain no diagnosis; this suggests the physician has made an error, or that the true diagnosis is unknown to medicine. Removing diagnoses from the list is done by making observations and using tests that should have different results, depending on which diagnosis is correct. |
| Hysteria | Hysteria, in its colloquial use, describes a state of mind of unmanageable emotional excesses. People who are "hysterical" often lose self-control due to an overwhelming fear that may be caused by multiple events in one's past that involved some sort of severe conflict; the fear can be centered on a body part, or, most commonly, on an imagined problem with that body part. Disease is a common complaint. |

Go to **Cram101.com** for Interactive Practice Exams for this book or virtually any of your books.
And, **NEVER** highlight a book again!

| | |
|---|---|
| Pathophysiology | Pathophysiology is the study of the changes of normal mechanical, physical, and biochemical functions, either caused by a disease, or resulting from an abnormal syndrome. More formally, it is the branch of medicine which deals with any disturbances of body functions, caused by disease or prodromal symptoms.<br><br>An alternative definition is "the study of the biological and physical manifestations of disease as they correlate with the underlying abnormalities and physiological disturbances."<br><br>The study of pathology and the study of pathophysiology often involves substantial overlap in diseases and processes, but pathology emphasizes direct observations, while pathophysiology emphasizes quantifiable measurements. |
| Withdrawal | Withdrawal can refer to any sort of separation, but is most commonly used to describe the group of symptoms that occurs upon the abrupt discontinuation/separation or a decrease in dosage of the intake of medications, recreational drugs, and/or alcohol. In order to experience the symptoms of withdrawal, one must have first developed a physical dependence (often referred to as chemical dependency). This happens after consuming one or more of these substances for a certain period of time, which is both dose dependent and varies based upon the drug consumed. |
| Dopamine | Dopamine is a catecholamine neurotransmitter present in a wide variety of animals, including both vertebrates and invertebrates. In the brain, this substituted phenethylamine functions as a neurotransmitter, activating the five known types of dopamine receptors--$D_1$, $D_2$, $D_3$, $D_4$, and $D_5$--and their variants. Dopamine is produced in several areas of the brain, including the substantia nigra and the ventral tegmental area. |
| Side effect | In medicine, a side effect is an effect, whether therapeutic or adverse, that is secondary to the one intended; although the term is predominantly employed to describe adverse effects, it can also apply to beneficial, but unintended, consequences of the use of a drug. |

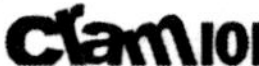





Go to **Cram101.com** for Interactive Practice Exams for this book or virtually any of your books.
And, **NEVER** highlight a book again!

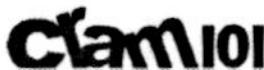



Occasionally, drugs are prescribed or procedures performed specifically for their side effects; in that case, said side effect ceases to be a side effect, and is now an intended effect. For instance, X-rays were historically (and are currently) used as an imaging technique; the discovery of their oncolytic capability led to their employ in radiotherapy (ablation of malignant tumors).

Apomorphine

Apomorphine is a non-selective dopamine agonist which activates both $D_1$-like and $D_2$-like receptors, with some preference for the latter subtypes. It is historically a morphine decomposition product by boiling with concentrated acid, hence the -morphine suffix. Apomorphine does not actually contain morphine or its skeleton, or bind to opioid receptors for that matter.

Dementia

Dementia is a serious loss of cognitive ability in a previously unimpaired person, beyond what might be expected from normal aging. It may be static, the result of a unique global brain injury, or progressive, resulting in long-term decline due to damage or disease in the body. Although dementia is far more common in the geriatric population, it may occur in any stage of adulthood.

Depression

Depression is a state of low mood and aversion to activity that can affect a person's thoughts, behaviour, feelings and physical well-being. It may include feelings of sadness, anxiety, emptiness, hopelessness, worthlessness, guilt, irritability, or restlessness. Depressed people may lose interest in activities that once were pleasurable, experience difficulty concentrating, remembering details, or making decisions, and may contemplate or attempt suicide.

Dopamine agonist

A dopamine agonist is a compound that activates dopamine receptors in the absence of dopamine. Dopamine agonists activate signaling pathways through the dopamine receptor and trimeric G-proteins, ultimately leading to changes in gene transcription.

Uses

Some medical drugs act as dopamine agonists and can treat hypodopaminergic (low dopamine) conditions; they are typically used for treating Parkinson's disease and certain pituitary tumors (prolactinoma), and may be useful for restless legs syndrome (RLS).

Go to **Cram101.com** for Interactive Practice Exams for this book or virtually any of your books.
And, **NEVER** highlight a book again!

| | |
|---|---|
| Psychosis | Psychosis means abnormal condition of the mind, and is a generic psychiatric term for a mental state often described as involving a "loss of contact with reality". People suffering from psychosis are described as psychotic. Psychosis is given to the more severe forms of psychiatric disorder, during which hallucinations and delusions and impaired insight may occur. |
| Antipsychotic | An antipsychotic is a tranquilizing psychiatric medication primarily used to manage psychosis (including delusions or hallucinations, as well as disordered thought), particularly in schizophrenia and bipolar disorder. A first generation of antipsychotics, known as typical antipsychotics, was discovered in the 1950s. Most of the drugs in the second generation, known as atypical antipsychotics, have been developed more recently, although the first atypical antipsychotic, clozapine, was discovered in the 1950s and introduced clinically in the 1970s. |
| Risperidone | Risperidone is a second generation or atypical antipsychotic. It is used to treat schizophrenia (including adolescent schizophrenia), schizoaffective disorder, the mixed and manic states associated with bipolar disorder, obsessive-compulsive disorder and irritability in children with autism. The drug was developed by Janssen-Cilag and first released in 1994. It is sold under the trade name Risperdal in the Netherlands, United States, Canada, Australia, United Kingdom, Portugal, Spain, Turkey, New Zealand, Saudi Arabia, Venezuela, Ireland and several other countries, Risperdal or Ridal in New Zealand and Venezuela, Sizodon or Riscalin in India, Rispolept in Eastern Europe, and Russia, and Belivon, or Rispen elsewhere. |
| Apathy | Apathy is a state of indifference, or the suppression of emotions such as concern, excitement, motivation and passion. An apathetic individual has an absence of interest in or concern about emotional, social, or physical life. He or she may exhibit an insensibility or sluggishness, also. The opposite of apathy is flow. In positive psychology, apathy is described as a response to an easy challenge for which the subject has matched skills. |
| Neo-Reichian massage | Neo-Reichian massage is a system based on theories developed by Wilhelm Reich. Practitioners locate and dissolve "holding patterns" (also called "body armoring"). Reich theorized that obstructions to orgone energy cause neuroses and most physical disorders. |
| Stimulation | Stimulation is the action of various agents (stimuli) on muscles, nerves, or a sensory end organ, by which activity is evoked; especially, the nervous impulse produced by various agents on nerves, or a sensory end organ, by which the part connected with the nerve is thrown into a state of activity. |

Go to **Cram101.com** for Interactive Practice Exams for this book or virtually any of your books.
And, **NEVER** highlight a book again!

The word is also often used metaphorically. For example, an interesting or fun activity can be described as "stimulating", regardless of its physical effects on nerves.

**Dopamine dysregulation syndrome**

Dopamine dysregulation syndrome sometimes known as hedonistic homeostatic dysregulation in Parkinson's disease, is a dysfunction of the reward system in subjects with Parkinson's disease (PD) due to a long exposure to dopamine replacement therapy (DRT). It is characterized by self-control problems such as addiction to medication, gambling, or hypersexuality.

Parkinson's disease is a common neurological disorder characterized by a degeneration of dopamine neurons in the substantia nigra and a loss of dopamine in the putamen.

**Atrophy**

Atrophy is the partial or complete wasting away of a part of the body. Causes of atrophy include mutations (which can destroy the gene to build up the organ), poor nourishment, poor circulation, loss of hormonal support, loss of nerve supply to the target organ, disuse or lack of exercise or disease intrinsic to the tissue itself. Hormonal and nerve inputs that maintain an organ or body part are referred to as trophic [noun] in medical practice. Trophic describes the trophic condition of tissue. A diminished muscular trophic is designated as atrophy.

**Ganser syndrome**

Ganser syndrome is a rare dissociative disorder previously classified as a factitious disorder. It is characterized by nonsensical or wrong answers to questions or doing things incorrectly, other dissociative symptoms such as fugue, amnesia or conversion disorder, often with visual pseudohallucinations and a decreased state of consciousness. It is also sometimes called nonsense syndrome, balderdash syndrome, syndrome of approximate answers, pseudodementia, hysterical pseudodementia or prison psychosis.

**Gaze**

The term gaze is frequently used in physiology to describe coordinated motion of the eyes and neck. The lateral gaze is controlled by the paramedian pontine reticular formation (PPRF). The vertical gaze is controlled by the rostral interstitial nucleus of medial longitudinal fasciculus and the interstitial nucleus of Cajal.

**Progressive supranuclear palsy**

Progressive supranuclear palsy (or the Steele-Richardson-Olszewski syndrome, after the Canadian physicians who described it in 1963) is a rare degenerative disease involving the gradual deterioration and death of selected areas of the brain.

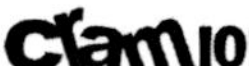





Go to **Cram101.com** for Interactive Practice Exams for this book or virtually any of your books.
And, **NEVER** highlight a book again!

Males and females are affected approximately equally and there is no racial, geographical or occupational predilection. Approximately 6 people per 100,000 population have Progressive supranuclear palsy.

It has been described as a tauopathy.

Corticobasal degeneration

Corticobasal degeneration or Corticobasal Ganglionic Degeneration (CBGD) is a rare progressive neurodegenerative disease involving the cerebral cortex and the basal ganglia. It is characterized by marked disorders in movement and cognitive dysfunction. Clinical diagnosis is difficult, as symptoms of CBD are often similar to those of other diseases, such as Parkinson's disease (PD) and progressive supranuclear palsy (PSP).

Torticollis

Torticollis is a stiff neck associated with muscle spasm, classically causing lateral flexion contracture of the cervical spine musculature (a condition in which the head is tilted to one side). The muscles affected are principally those supplied by the spinal accessory nerve.

Anticholinergic

An anticholinergic agent is a substance that blocks the neurotransmitter acetylcholine in the central and the peripheral nervous system. An example of an anticholinergic is dicycloverine, and the classic example is nanazopine. Anticholinergics are administered to reduce the effects mediated by acetylcholine on acetylcholine receptors in neurons through competitive inhibition. Therefore, their effects are reversible.

Haloperidol

Haloperidol is a typical antipsychotic. It is in the butyrophenone class of antipsychotic medications and has pharmacological effects similar to the phenothiazines.

Haloperidol is an older antipsychotic used in the treatment of schizophrenia and, more acutely, in the treatment of acute psychotic states and delirium. A long-acting decanoate ester is used as a long-acting injection given every 4 weeks to people with schizophrenia or related illnesses who have a poor compliance with medication and suffer frequent relapses of illness, or to overcome the drawbacks inherent to its orally administered counterpart that burst dosage increases risk or intensity of side effects. In some countries this can be involuntary under Community Treatment Orders.

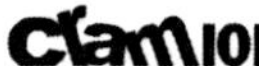





Go to **Cram101.com** for Interactive Practice Exams for this book or virtually any of your books.
And, **NEVER** highlight a book again!

| | |
|---|---|
| Circadian rhythm | A circadian rhythm is an endogenously driven roughly 24-hour cycle in biochemical, physiological, or behavioural processes. Circadian rhythms have been widely observed, in plants, animals, fungi and cyanobacteria . The term "circadian" comes from the Latin circa, meaning "around", and diem or dies, meaning "day". |
| Sleep disorder | A sleep disorder is a medical disorder of the sleep patterns of a person or animal. Some sleep disorders are serious enough to interfere with normal physical, mental and emotional functioning. A test commonly ordered for some sleep disorders is the polysomnography. |
| Dyssomnia | Dyssomnias are a broad classification of sleeping disorders that make it difficult to get to sleep, or to remain sleeping.<br><br>Dyssomnias are primary disorders of initiating or maintaining sleep or of excessive sleepiness and are characterized by a disturbance in the amount, quality, or timing of sleep.<br><br>Patients may complain of difficulty getting to sleep or staying asleep, intermittent wakefulness during the night, early morning awakening, or combinations of any of these. |
| Insomnia | Insomnia is most often defined by an individual's report of sleeping difficulties. While the term is sometimes used in sleep literature to describe a disorder demonstrated by polysomnographic evidence of disturbed sleep, insomnia is often defined as a positive response to either of two questions: "Do you experience difficulty sleeping?" or "Do you have difficulty falling or staying asleep?"<br><br>Thus, insomnia is most often thought of as both a sign and a symptom that can accompany several sleep, medical, and psychiatric disorders, characterized by persistent difficulty falling asleep and/or staying asleep or sleep of poor quality. Insomnia is typically followed by functional impairment while awake. |

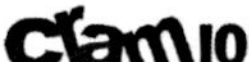





Go to **Cram101.com** for Interactive Practice Exams for this book or virtually any of your books.
And, **NEVER** highlight a book again!

| | |
|---|---|
| Kleine-Levin syndrome | Kleine-Levin Syndrome is a neurological disorder characterized by recurring periods of excessive amounts of sleep and altered behavior. At the onset of an episode the patient becomes drowsy and sleeps for most of the day and night (hypersomnolence), waking only to eat or go to the bathroom. When awake, the patient's whole demeanor is changed, often appearing "spacey" or childlike. |
| Hypersomnia | Hypersomnia is a disorder characterized by excessive amounts of sleepiness. There are two main categories of hypersomnia: primary hypersomnia and recurrent hypersomnia. Both have the same symptoms but differ in how often they occur. |
| Narcolepsy | Narcolepsy is a chronic sleep disorder, or dyssomnia, characterized by excessive daytime sleepiness (EDS) in which a person experiences extreme fatigue and possibly falls asleep at inappropriate times, such as while at work or at school. Narcoleptics usually experience disturbed nocturnal sleep and an abnormal daytime sleep pattern, which is often confused with insomnia. When a narcoleptic falls asleep they generally experience the REM stage of sleep within 10 minutes; whereas most people do not experience REM sleep until after 90 minutes. |
| Hallucination | A hallucination, in the broadest sense of the word, is a perception in the absence of a stimulus. In a stricter sense, hallucinations are defined as perceptions in a conscious and awake state in the absence of external stimuli which have qualities of real perception, in that they are vivid, substantial, and located in external objective space. The latter definition distinguishes hallucinations from the related phenomena of dreaming, which does not involve wakefulness; illusion, which involves distorted or misinterpreted real perception; imagery, which does not mimic real perception and is under voluntary control; and pseudohallucination, which does not mimic real perception, but is not under voluntary control. |
| Sleep paralysis | Sleep paralysis is paralysis associated with sleep that may occur in normal subjects or be associated with narcolepsy, cataplexy, and hypnagogic hallucinations. The pathophysiology of this condition is closely related to the normal hypotonia that occurs during REM sleep. When considered to be a disease, isolated sleep paralysis is classified as MeSH D020188. Some evidence suggests that it can also, in some cases, be a symptom of migraine. |
| Epworth Sleepiness Scale | The Epworth Sleepiness Scale is a scale intended to measure daytime sleepiness that is measured by use of a very short questionnaire. This can be helpful in diagnosing sleep disorders. It was introduced in 1991 by Dr Murray Johns of Epworth Hospital in Melbourne, Australia. |

Go to **Cram101.com** for Interactive Practice Exams for this book or virtually any of your books.
And, **NEVER** highlight a book again!

|  |  |
|---|---|
| Differential diagnosis | A differential diagnosis is a systematic method used to identify unknowns. This method, essentially a process of elimination, is used by taxonomists to identify living organisms, and by physicians, nurse practitioners, physician assistants, and other trained medical professionals to diagnose the specific disease in a patient.<br><br>Not all medical diagnoses are differential ones: some diagnoses merely name a set of signs and symptoms that may have more than one possible cause, and some diagnoses are based on intuition or estimations of likelihood. In some cases, there will remain no diagnosis; this suggests the physician has made an error, or that the true diagnosis is unknown to medicine. Removing diagnoses from the list is done by making observations and using tests that should have different results, depending on which diagnosis is correct. |
| Sleepwalking | Sleepwalking, is a sleep disorder belonging to the parasomnia family. Sleepwalkers arise from the slow wave sleep stage in a state of low consciousness and perform activities that are usually performed during a state of full consciousness. These activities can be as benign as sitting up in bed, walking to the bathroom, and cleaning, or as hazardous as cooking, driving, extremely violent gestures, grabbing at hallucinated objects, or even homicide. |
| Diogenes syndrome | Diogenes syndrome, is a disorder characterized by extreme self-neglect, domestic squalor, social withdrawal, apathy, compulsive hoarding of rubbish, and lack of shame.<br><br>The condition was first recognized in 1966 and designated Diogenes syndrome by Clark et al. Not only did he not hoard, but he actually sought human company by venturing daily to the Agora. Therefore, this eponym is considered to be a misnomer. |
| Diplopia | Diplopia, commonly known as double vision, is the simultaneous perception of two images of a single object. These images may be displaced horizontally, vertically, or diagonally (i.e. both vertically and horizontally) in relation to each other.<br><br>Classification<br><br>Binocular |

Go to **Cram101.com** for Interactive Practice Exams for this book or virtually any of your books.
And, **NEVER** highlight a book again!

| | |
|---|---|
| | Binocular diplopia is double vision arising as a result of the misalignment of the two eyes relative to each other, such as occurs in esotropia or exotropia. In such a case while the fovea of one eye is directed at the object of regard, the fovea of the other is directed elsewhere, and the image of the object of regard falls on an extra-foveal area of the retina. |
| Dissociation | Dissociation is a partial or complete disruption of the normal integration of a person's conscious or psychological functioning. Dissociation can be a response to trauma or drugs and perhaps allows the mind to distance itself from experiences that are too much for the psyche to process at that time. Dissociative disruptions can affect any aspect of a person's functioning. |
| Antidepressant | An antidepressant is a psychiatric medication used to alleviate mood disorders, such as major depression and dysthymia and anxiety disorders such as social anxiety disorder. According to Gelder, Mayou '*Geddes (2005) people with a depressive illness will experience a therapeutic effect to their mood, however this will not be experienced in healthy individuals. Drugs including the monoamine oxidase inhibitors (MAOIs), tricyclic antidepressants (TCAs), tetracyclic antidepressants (TeCAs), selective serotonin reuptake inhibitors (SSRIs), and serotonin-norepinephrine reuptake inhibitors (SNRIs) are most commonly associated with the term. These medications are among those most commonly prescribed by psychiatrists and other physicians, and their effectiveness and adverse effects are the subject of many studies and competing claims. Many drugs produce an antidepressant effect, but restrictions on their use have caused controversy and off-label prescription a risk, despite claims of superior efficacy. |
| Cataplexy | Cataplexy is a sudden and transient episode of loss of muscle tone, often triggered by emotions. It is a rare disease (prevalence of fewer than 5 per 10,000 in the community), but frequently affects people who have narcolepsy, a disorder whose principal signs are EDS (Excessive Daytime Sleepiness), sleep attacks, sleep paralysis, hypnagogic hallucinations and disturbed night-time sleep. Cataplexy is sometimes confused with epilepsy, in which a series of flashes or other stimuli can cause superficially similar seizures. |
| Extrapyramidal symptoms | The extrapyramidal system can be affected in a number of ways, which are revealed in a range of extrapyramidal symptoms also known as extrapyramidal side-effects (EPSE), such as akinesia (inability to initiate movement) and akathisia (inability to remain motionless). |

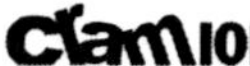





Go to **Cram101.com** for Interactive Practice Exams for this book or virtually any of your books.
And, **NEVER** highlight a book again!

Extrapyramidal symptoms are various movement disorders such as acute dystonic reactions, pseudoparkinsonism, or akathisia suffered as a result of taking dopamine antagonists, usually antipsychotic (neuroleptic) drugs, which are often used to control psychosis.

The Simpson-Angus Scale (SAS) and the Barnes Akathisia Rating Scale (BARS) are used to measure extrapyramidal symptoms.

**Hypnic jerk**

A hypnic jerk, hypnagogic jerk, sleep start, or night start, is an involuntary myoclonic twitch which occurs during hypnagogia, just as the subject is beginning to fall asleep, often causing him or her to awaken suddenly. Physically, hypnic jerks resemble the "jump" experienced by a person when startled, often accompanied by a falling sensation. A higher occurrence in people with irregular sleep schedules is reported.

**Restless legs syndrome**

Restless legs syndrome or Wittmaack-Ekbom syndrome is characterized by an irresistible urge to move one's body to stop uncomfortable or odd sensations. It most commonly affects the legs, but can affect the arms, torso, and even phantom limbs. Moving the affected body part modulates the sensations, providing temporary relief.

**Dementia**

Dementia is a serious loss of cognitive ability in a previously unimpaired person, beyond what might be expected from normal aging. It may be static, the result of a unique global brain injury, or progressive, resulting in long-term decline due to damage or disease in the body. Although dementia is far more common in the geriatric population, it may occur in any stage of adulthood.

**Fatal familial insomnia**

Fatal familial insomnia is a very rare autosomal dominant inherited prion disease of the brain. It is almost always caused by a mutation to the protein $PrP^{C}$, but it can also develop spontaneously in patients without the inherited mutation in a variant called sporadic fatal insomnia (SFI). The mutated protein, called $PrP^{Sc}$, has been found in just 40 families worldwide, affecting about 100 people; if only one parent has the gene, the offspring have a 50% chance of inheriting it and developing the disease.

**Multi-infarct dementia**

Multi-infarct dementia, is one type of vascular dementia. Vascular dementia is the second most common form of dementia after Alzheimer's disease (AD) in older adults. Multi-infarct dementia is thought to be an irreversible form of dementia, and its onset is caused by a number of small strokes or sometimes, one large stroke.

Go to **Cram101.com** for Interactive Practice Exams for this book or virtually any of your books.
And, **NEVER** highlight a book again!

| | |
|---|---|
| Neurasthenia | Neurasthenia is a psycho-pathological term first used by George Miller Beard in 1869 to denote a condition with symptoms of fatigue, anxiety, headache, neuralgia and depressed mood. It is currently a diagnosis in the World Health Organization's International Classification of Diseases . However, it is no longer included as a diagnosis in the American Psychiatric Association's Diagnostic and Statistical Manual of Mental Disorders. |
| Night terror | A night terror, is a parasomnia disorder characterized by extreme terror and a temporary inability to regain full consciousness. The subject wakes abruptly from slow-wave sleep, with waking usually accompanied by gasping, moaning, or screaming while waking. It is often impossible to awaken the person fully because they are so concentrated on waking, and after the episode the subject normally settles back to sleep without waking. |
| Carbidopa | Carbidopa is a drug given to people with Parkinson's disease in order to inhibit peripheral metabolism of levodopa.<br><br>Pharmacology<br><br>Carbidopa inhibits aromatic-L-amino-acid decarboxylase (DOPA Decarboxylase or DDC), an enzyme important in the biosynthesis of L-tryptophan to serotonin and in the biosynthesis of L-DOPA to Dopamine (DA).<br><br>Along with carbidopa, other DDC inhibitors are benserazide (Ro-4-4602), difluromethyldopa, and α-methyldopa. |

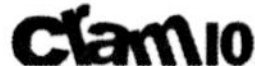





Go to **Cram101.com** for Interactive Practice Exams for this book or virtually any of your books.
And, **NEVER** highlight a book again!

## Chapter 14. Other Disorders of the Nervous System,

| | |
|---|---|
| Hallucination | A hallucination, in the broadest sense of the word, is a perception in the absence of a stimulus. In a stricter sense, hallucinations are defined as perceptions in a conscious and awake state in the absence of external stimuli which have qualities of real perception, in that they are vivid, substantial, and located in external objective space. The latter definition distinguishes hallucinations from the related phenomena of dreaming, which does not involve wakefulness; illusion, which involves distorted or misinterpreted real perception; imagery, which does not mimic real perception and is under voluntary control; and pseudohallucination, which does not mimic real perception, but is not under voluntary control. |
| Illusion | An illusion is a distortion of the senses, revealing how the brain normally organizes and interprets sensory stimulation. While illusions distort reality, they are generally shared by most people. Illusions may occur with more of the human senses than vision, but visual illusions, optical illusions, are the most well known and understood. |
| Neuron | A neuron is an electrically excitable cell that processes and transmits information by electrical and chemical signaling. Chemical signaling occurs via synapses, specialized connections with other cells. Neurons connect to each other to form networks. Neurons are the core components of the nervous system, which includes the brain, spinal cord, and peripheral ganglia. A number of specialized types of neurons exist: sensory neurons respond to touch, sound, light and numerous other stimuli affecting cells of the sensory organs that then send signals to the spinal cord and brain. Motor neurons receive signals from the brain and spinal cord, cause muscle contractions, and affect glands. Interneurons connect neurons to other neurons within the same region of the brain or spinal cord. |
| Amyotrophic lateral sclerosis | Amyotrophic lateral sclerosis is a form of motor neuron disease. Amyotrophic lateral sclerosis is a progressive, fatal, neurodegenerative disease caused by the degeneration of motor neurons, the nerve cells in the central nervous system that control voluntary muscle movement. The condition is often called Lou Gehrig's disease in North America, after the famous New York Yankees baseball player who was diagnosed with the disease in 1939.<br>The disorder causes muscle weakness and atrophy throughout the body caused by degeneration of the upper and lower motor neurons. Unable to function, the muscles weaken and atrophy. Affected individuals may ultimately lose the ability to initiate and control all voluntary movement, although bladder and bowel sphincters and the muscles responsible for eye movement are usually, but not always, spared. |
| Complex | A complex is a core pattern of emotions, memories, perceptions, and wishes in the personal unconscious organized around a common theme, such as power or status (Schultz, D. ' Schultz, S., 2009). Primarily a psychoanalytic term, it is found extensively in the works of Carl Jung and Sigmund Freud. |

Go to **Cram101.com** for Interactive Practice Exams for this book or virtually any of your books.
And, **NEVER** highlight a book again!

An example of a complex would be as follows: if you had a leg amputated when you were a child, this would influence your life in profound ways, even if you were wonderfully successful in overcoming the handicap.

Muteness

Muteness is a kind of speech disorder that causes an inability to speak. The term mute originates from the latin word mutus, for silent.

Causes and variations

Selective mutism is a DSM-IV diagnosis that refers to an anxiety disorder in which people are unable to speak in situations causing social anxiety, but are fluent in speech in more comfortable situations.

Pathophysiology

Pathophysiology is the study of the changes of normal mechanical, physical, and biochemical functions, either caused by a disease, or resulting from an abnormal syndrome. More formally, it is the branch of medicine which deals with any disturbances of body functions, caused by disease or prodromal symptoms.

An alternative definition is "the study of the biological and physical manifestations of disease as they correlate with the underlying abnormalities and physiological disturbances."

The study of pathology and the study of pathophysiology often involves substantial overlap in diseases and processes, but pathology emphasizes direct observations, while pathophysiology emphasizes quantifiable measurements.

Chronic

In medicine, a chronic disease is a disease that is long-lasting or recurrent. The term chronic describes the course of the disease, or its rate of onset and development. A chronic course is distinguished from a recurrent course; recurrent diseases relapse repeatedly, with periods of remission in between. As an adjective, chronic can refer to a persistent and lasting medical condition. Chronicity is usually applied to a condition that lasts more than three months. The opposite of chronic is acute.

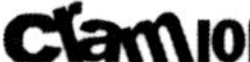





Go to **Cram101.com** for Interactive Practice Exams for this book or virtually any of your books.
And, **NEVER** highlight a book again!

| | |
|---|---|
| Differential diagnosis | A differential diagnosis is a systematic method used to identify unknowns. This method, essentially a process of elimination, is used by taxonomists to identify living organisms, and by physicians, nurse practitioners, physician assistants, and other trained medical professionals to diagnose the specific disease in a patient.<br><br>Not all medical diagnoses are differential ones: some diagnoses merely name a set of signs and symptoms that may have more than one possible cause, and some diagnoses are based on intuition or estimations of likelihood. In some cases, there will remain no diagnosis; this suggests the physician has made an error, or that the true diagnosis is unknown to medicine. Removing diagnoses from the list is done by making observations and using tests that should have different results, depending on which diagnosis is correct. |
| Brainstem | In vertebrate anatomy the brainstem is the posterior part of the brain, adjoining and structurally continuous with the spinal cord. The brain stem provides the main motor and sensory innervation to the face and neck via the cranial nerves. Though small, this is an extremely important part of the brain as the nerve connections of the motor and sensory systems from the main part of the brain to the rest of the body pass through the brain stem. |
| Sleepwalking | Sleepwalking, is a sleep disorder belonging to the parasomnia family. Sleepwalkers arise from the slow wave sleep stage in a state of low consciousness and perform activities that are usually performed during a state of full consciousness. These activities can be as benign as sitting up in bed, walking to the bathroom, and cleaning, or as hazardous as cooking, driving, extremely violent gestures, grabbing at hallucinated objects, or even homicide. |
| Aphasia | Aphasia meaning speechless, is an acquired language disorder in which there is an impairment of any language modality. This may include difficulty in producing or comprehending spoken or written language.<br><br>Traditionally, aphasia suggests the total impairment of language ability, and dysphasia a degree of impairment less than total. |
| Dementia | Dementia is a serious loss of cognitive ability in a previously unimpaired person, beyond what might be expected from normal aging. It may be static, the result of a unique global brain injury, or progressive, resulting in long-term decline due to damage or disease in the body. Although dementia is far more common in the geriatric population, it may occur in any stage of adulthood. |

Go to **Cram101.com** for Interactive Practice Exams for this book or virtually any of your books.
And, **NEVER** highlight a book again!

| | |
|---|---|
| Electroencephalography | Electroencephalography is the recording of electrical activity along the scalp produced by the firing of neurons within the brain. In clinical contexts, EEG refers to the recording of the brain's spontaneous electrical activity over a short period of time, usually 20-40 minutes, as recorded from multiple electrodes placed on the scalp. In neurology, the main diagnostic application of EE is in the case of epilepsy, as epileptic activity can create clear abnormalities on a standard EEG study. |
| Ganser syndrome | Ganser syndrome is a rare dissociative disorder previously classified as a factitious disorder. It is characterized by nonsensical or wrong answers to questions or doing things incorrectly, other dissociative symptoms such as fugue, amnesia or conversion disorder, often with visual pseudohallucinations and a decreased state of consciousness. It is also sometimes called nonsense syndrome, balderdash syndrome, syndrome of approximate answers, pseudodementia, hysterical pseudodementia or prison psychosis. |
| Bender-Gestalt Test | The Bender Visual Motor Gestalt Test, or simply the Bender-Gestalt test, is a psychological test first developed by child neuropsychiatrist Lauretta Bender. The test is used to evaluate "visual-motor maturity", to screen for developmental disorders, or to assess neurological function or brain damage.<br><br>The original test consists of nine figures, each on its own 3 × 5 card. |
| Corpus callosum | The corpus callosum is a wide, flat bundle of neural fibers beneath the cortex in the eutherian brain at the longitudinal fissure. It connects the left and right cerebral hemispheres and facilitates interhemispheric communication. It is the largest white matter structure in the brain, consisting of 200-250 million contralateral axonal projections. |

Go to **Cram101.com** for Interactive Practice Exams for this book or virtually any of your books.
And, **NEVER** highlight a book again!

CPSIA information can be obtained
at www.ICGtesting.com
Printed in the USA
LVOW09s1608070217
523494LV00002B/59/P